Diab
and

The Exorcist

Diabolical Possession and the Case Behind *The Exorcist*

An Overview of Scientific Research with Interviews with Witnesses and Experts

SERGIO A. RUEDA

Foreword by STANLEY KRIPPNER

McFarland & Company, Inc., Publishers
Jefferson, North Carolina

LIBRARY OF CONGRESS CATALOGUING-IN-PUBLICATION DATA

Names: Rueda, Sergio A., author.
Title: Diabolical possession and the case behind the exorcist : an
    overview of scientific research with interviews with witnesses
    and experts / Sergio A. Rueda ; foreword by Stanley Krippner.
Description: Jefferson, North Carolina : McFarland & Company, Inc.,
    Publishers, 2018. | Includes bibliographical references and index.
Identifiers: LCCN 2018040723 | ISBN 9781476673844 (softcover : acid
    free paper) ∞
Subjects: LCSH: Demoniac possession. | Exorcism. | Doe, Roland.
Classification: LCC BF1555 .R84 2018 | DDC 133.4/26—dc23
LC record available at https://lccn.loc.gov/2018040723Identifiers:

BRITISH LIBRARY CATALOGUING DATA ARE AVAILABLE

ISBN (print) 978-1-4766-7384-4
ISBN (ebook) 978-1-4766-3251-3

Front cover: Linda Blair in The *Exorcist*, 1973 (Warner Bros.
Pictures/Photofest)

Printed in the United States of America

McFarland & Company, Inc., Publishers
    Box 611, Jefferson, North Carolina 28640
    www.mcfarlandpub.com

With love and recognition to Anne Carrol,
my mother Antonia, sister Erika,
son José and mentors Stanley Krippner,
Carlos Alvarado and Ignacio Arróniz

"The evil in this world that we have to deal with, is, and this I mean deliberately, to refer that exorcism is not evil out there that impinges upon us, it's the evil in our hearts. And our job in life is to drive out that evil, the internal evil, the habitual evil, the evil we don't even recognize, and replace it with the gentle, loving, kindly philosophy of life that is interested in being there for other people."
—Fr. Frank Bober, 1996, documentary *In the Grip of Evil*

Table of Contents

Acknowledgments

I am grateful to the following people and organizations for their support, valuable editorial assistance, logistical and financial support, and motivation to complete this book:

The Parapsychology Foundation of New York City for providing the funds for the field research into the case on which this book is based. This financial support allowed me to interview actual participants in the real events.

Dr. Stanley Krippner, my primary mentor, who supervised my doctoral dissertation on "Medical-Psychological Approaches to the Mount Rainier Exorcism," and also guided me in my studies throughout my doctoral program. In addition, Dr. Krippner encouraged me to present this dissertation at the 49th Annual Scientific Parapsychological Association Convention held in Stockholm, Sweden, August 4–6, 2006.

Drs. Carlos S. Alvarado and Nancy Zingrone, mentors with regard to my doctoral dissertation and for their valuable editorial assistance and academic guidance in completing this research project.

Anne Carrol: Former business manager of Duke Parapsychology Laboratory, who assisted me in the location of key documents on the Mount Rainier Exorcism, such as the Jesuit Report and the old correspondence of Dr. J.B. Rhine at the archives of the Laboratory.

Drs. Richard Broughton, K. Ramakrishna Rao and John Krueger, researcher, former director, and director at the Foundation for Research on the Nature of Man and Rhine Research Center in Durham, North Carolina, for granting me special permissions to consult and access the confidential archives of the Foundation and the archives of the former Duke Parapsychology Laboratory related to the case on which William Peter Blatty based *The Exorcist*.

The Reverend Luther and Ruth Schulze for their kindness and very helpful interviews for this book.

Ida Mae Donley for providing me with a copy of the Jesuit Report and her assistance to visit the original places in which the Mount Rainier Exorcism took place.

Robert L. Henninger, president and CEO of Henninger Media Services, Inc., for providing me with the permission to use the transcripts and quotations of some of the interviews in the documentary *In the Grip of Evil* to complement the information in this book.

Ignacio Arroniz, MD, for his enormous financial support at the personal and organizational level to our institute of medicine, which allowed me sufficient time to complete the research and book projects.

Enrique Soto Canales, MD, director of Hospital Poliplaza Médica in Juarez, México, who provided financial support to our institute of medicine so that I could take a leave of absence to complete this book.

Foreword
by Stanley Krippner, Ph.D.

In 1971 a novel by William Peter Blatty was published and became a best-seller. *The Exorcist* tells the story of the alleged demonic possession of a young girl and the efforts of two priests to "exorcise" or expel the demon. Few readers knew that the idea for the novel came to Blatty when he was a student at Georgetown University, where he heard an account of an exorcism performed by a Jesuit priest who worked with a young boy in Maryland who he felt was afflicted by demonic forces.

In 2011, Blatty published a 40th anniversary edition of *The Exorcist*, which included some new and revised material including an additional character. Earlier, William Peter Blatty had written *Legion*, a sequel to the original book, and in 2012 a stage adaptation was performed, followed by a radio adaptation for the BBC in 2014.

Perhaps the version that reached the largest number of people was the 1973 film, *The Exorcist*, which won William Peter Blatty an Academy Award for Best Adapted Screenplay, and which—over four decades later—has grossed some $500 million in worldwide sales on an original budget of $11 million. There were several cinematic sequels and prequels, of varying degrees of quality, and a television series in 2016 that had little in common with the earlier film, except for its title.

Shortly after Warner Brothers acquired the rights to the book, I was sitting alone in my office at Maimonides Medical Center in Brooklyn, New York. By chance, I was working overtime or would have missed my surprise visitor. Responding to a knock on my door, I welcomed William Friedkin, who had been named director of the forthcoming film. William Friedkin introduced himself, almost apologetically, but I told him that I had admired two of his earlier films, *The Boys in the Band* and *The French Connection*, for the latter of which he had won the Academy Award for best director.

William Friedkin had heard of my parapsychological research and wanted to discuss the approach he should take with his new project. I had not read *The Exorcist* but was familiar with the story, so told him: "Mr. Friedkin, I can see two approaches you could take to the project. One would resemble the classic Japanese film *Rashomon*. You will recall that the movie focuses on a murder, but is told in four different ways, one by the murderer, one by the wife of the victim, one by the spirit of the victim, and one by an eyewitness. Your film could do the same: one version by the afflicted girl, one by her mother, one by the exorcist, and one by the demon—who is actually a 'devil's advocate' maintaining that he was constructed by the imagination, fears, and attention-getting strategies of the victim herself. This approach would win plaudits from the critics but would leave many viewers unsatisfied because the solution to the alleged possession is left up to them. The alternative would be to accept the existence of the demon as being literally true, and move forward from there. This version may not win over the critics, but it will make a fortune at the box office."

William Friedkin and I discussed other aspects of the film, including his desire to cast a young "psychic" as Regan, the afflicted girl. I suggested that he opt for a professional actress, but did give him the name of a girl who had performed well in our parapsychology experiments. He actually visited the girl and her mother, who asked, "Will my daughter be required to do everything that is in the book, such as masturbating with a crucifix?" When Friedkin answered affirmatively, she retorted, "I would never allow my daughter to be in such a movie." Her daughter was crushed and would not speak to her mother for a week. Friedkin ended up casting Linda Blair, who did an exemplary job as Regan, winning a Golden Globe Award as best supporting actress.

When the film was released it received mixed reviews, as I had predicted. However, its stature has grown over the years, and it is now considered one of the best films in the horror genre. *Empire Magazine* included it in its list of the 500 greatest films ever made, and it also appears in the *New York Times* list of the 1000 best films of all time. Shortly after the film's release, a friend of mine met William Friedkin at a Hollywood party and asked if he remembered meeting me. According to my friend, Friedkin replied, "I could never have made *The Exorcist* the way I did without Dr. Krippner's advice."

Little did I know that decades later I would be supervising Sergio A. Rueda's doctoral dissertation on the real-life events that preceded William Peter Blatty's novel and William Friedkin's movie. A 1993 book by Thomas B. Allen had documented the case using the original exorcist's notes as well as the testimony of another priest who was an eyewitness observer of the priest's attempts to expel demonic forces from the young boy. Dr. Sergio Antonio Rueda turned his dissertation into this book, and it includes even more material, including documents and interviews that he collected over a period of several years, as well as information gleaned during several site visits. Dr. Rueda also presents several interpretations of the actual events, *Rashomon*-style, before sharing his own conclusions with his readers.

Dr. Rueda's book is filled with suspense of its own, taking its reader from one perspective to another, slowly filling in gaps and fitting pieces of the puzzle together. The result is an engrossing account that occupies a unique niche in the ongoing saga of a child whose reported experiences present challenges to established ways of viewing the world and its inhabitants. It is to Dr. Rueda's credit that he takes a scientific approach to the enigma, carefully collecting data without preconceptions, allowing a factual narrative to emerge that is both entertaining and enlightening. The readers of this remarkable book will be puzzled and intrigued, and some may be offended—but they will never be bored.

Stanley Krippner is the past president of divisions 30-Hypnosis and 32-Humanistic Psychology of the American Psychological Association and winner of the association's Distinguished Contributions to the International Advancement of Psychology award of 2002.

Preface

In late 1973, women and men were lined up for blocks in the United States, and in many other countries around the world a year later. They were standing in line waiting to see a film. People were known to become ill watching it. Some fainted. Some ran out of the theater in tears. There were reports of people having to be institutionalized, and at least one miscarriage was attributed to viewing it. No, it wasn't a Beatles concert. It was a film called *The Exorcist*. The most terrifying film in the history of moviemaking, its success went beyond the expectations of the producers. The novel, which was a mega-bestseller, itself sold 13 million copies in the United States alone, and the movie was nominated for 10 Oscars.

At the present, William Friedkin's film continues to be a cult movie for those who feel called to ponder on the classic issues of good and evil. Many continue to investigate *The Exorcist* and the case on which it was based. Some tourists and investigative reporters even visit the places, not only where the movie was filmed, but where the original case took place. New television series based on *The Exorcist* appear from time to time, such as the one produced by Fox recently. Why does this fascination with *The Exorcist* continue even up to the present time? Sociologists have tried to explain the phenomenon as the result of the continuous presence in the world of good and evil. *The Exorcist* is the exact portrayal of this eternal battle that has influenced every society and its moral development.

Therefore, any additional information that may arise about the true case that served as the basis of the book and movie continues to spark interest in the media and the general public, as well as theologians and scholars in the field of demonology. This book reveals hidden information that remained unknown for many years, and it will shed surprising light on what really happened in the actual Mount Rainier Exorcism, the basis of *The Exorcist*. New documents have appeared, such as the Jesuit Report on the Mount Rainier case, and interviews of critical participants in the case will finally settle its real nature in the framework of science.

4

The book addresses the following issues: "Is demonic possession, like sin, one of the dead metaphors supposedly killed off by the scientific spirit of the 21st century?" "Is our quest for the existence of such phenomena reflected in the human need to live in a world where evil embodies the image of Satan—the fallen angel who inhabits the inner circle of Dante's inferno?" "Is the Antichrist a living force at work in our lives, awaiting his next opportunity to exert his influence as he attempts to drag the world into a state of chaos?" I will try to answer some of the above questions in the context of the most famous case in the history of Christianity on demonic possession and exorcism, the case known as the Mount Rainier exorcism, which took place in 1949 and was used by William Peter Blatty to write the novel *The Exorcist* and later the screenplay of the film.

Almost 50 years have passed since the novel and film were released in the early 1970s, but the number-one ranked horror movie in history still turns heads in the 21st century. However, before we explain why *The Exorcist* still impacts society at the present time, it is important to note that up until the early 1970s, before the movie was released, the ideas of demonic possession, exorcism and even the existence of the Devil, for the majority of the Catholic believers and society overall, were abstract ideas, popular beliefs that had no tangible evidence. For many experts in the fields of mental health and sociology, and even some religious leaders, they were myths consigned to the Middle Ages and to the books on the history of psychiatry and religion.

For many scholars in the fields of theology, sociology and mental health in the 20th century, the tendency was to move away from the idea of the Devil or actual demons, and write off Satan as a manufactured idea of the medieval church. They were considered literary constructs used by Jesus Christ as a metaphor to explain the concept of evil to his uneducated Jewish followers. For some modern psychiatrists, the terms demon and demonic possession were pre-Freudian terms used as figures of speech to explain mental illness at the time.

However, a cultural revolution on the ideas about demons, demonic possession and exorcism exploded with the movie *The Exorcist*. The film gave new life to Satan and his legions; the Devil now acquired a tangible existence, the demons became real, they spoke and interacted with humans and had to be fought and driven out of a possessed individual. Many of us had been taught as children, by religious authorities and our parents, about the eternal fight between good and evil in order to reinforce our moral, religious and social values. Now, we could be reminded of these moral values in the context of an extreme dramatized struggle in a film, with shocking images such as a statue of the Virgin at a church vandalized by the addition of an artificial penis. Also, the possessed girl in the movie, played by Linda Blair, manifests incredible feats of a supernatural nature and desecration, such as when she turns her head completely backwards and sticks a crucifix in her vagina during the exorcism.

Many moviegoers could not stand these horrible images, and walked out on the film in many cinemas around the world. Some of them were taken into ambulances stationed outside of the cinemas and even warranted psychiatric treatment. The impact of the movie brought renewed attention to the topic of demonic possession and exorcism in the modern era, and William Peter Blatty won an Academy Award for best adapted screenplay. Even at the present time, almost half a century after the movie was first released, interest in demonic possession and exorcism in our modern society continues. Filmmakers, companies specializing in scientific documentaries, and producers of television series, have continued to fill this interest and meet the need of many humans to understand the fight between good and evil in our modern society. For instance, in 1997 a dramatic documentary on the actual case on which William Peter Blatty based *The Exorcist* was produced by Henninger Media, titled *In the Grip of Evil*. Moreover, recently a successful television sequel was put out by Fox Television in 2016, loosely based on the William Peter Blatty novel. The series was so successful that it was renewed for 2017.

Clearly many members of society are hungry to understand this battle of good and evil, in order to learn how to get away from evil and lead a moral life in a corrupt and dangerous world. Interestingly, they still want to portray this battle in the framework of the story of *The Exorcist*. Back in the early 1970s, many people who viewed the movie, and experts on demonic possession and exorcism, knew that Williams Peter Blatty's *Exorcist* had been based on an actual case that had taken place in 1949 in Prince Georges County, Maryland. The fact that the movie had been based on an actual case made moviegoers curious about the real story. If the events narrated in the film were accurate and truthful about the real story, this film would reflect the real actions and influence of the demons in the world. It would also confirm and strengthen the audience's faith and beliefs in the dogmas of demonic possession and exorcism, as well as their belief in the existence of a superior being.

As a result, many reporters and researchers for many years underwent the trip to the area where the case had taken place, in order to find out the truth behind it. However, those involved in the original case, such as religious authorities and the very few witnesses who were still alive, refused to talk about the case. Also, the records of the exorcism had been hidden by the Catholic priests who conducted the exorcism.

The *Washington Post* had published concisely, in 1949, part of the story of a 14-year-old boy possessed by a demon on which *The Exorcist* was based. However, very little had become public of what really happened. Now the actual case can be better understood as a result of an extensive detailed account that has now emerged: the Jesuit Report, a document found hidden in the archives of the most prestigious institution dedicated to the investigation of paranormal phenomena, the Foundation for Research on the Nature of Man, formerly the Duke Parapsychology Laboratory. This document was found by coincidence by the author.

The Jesuit Report constitutes the most complete written account of a real demonic possession and exorcism case in the history of the church known up to the present time. This document, along with some extensive correspondence between the most prestigious parapsychologist of Duke University Parapsychology Laboratory and a skeptical Lutheran reverend involved in the case, here joins interviews from original witnesses, who were eager to speak of the case for the first time to the author. They will reveal some of the most amazing phenomena of a presumed supernatural nature in the Mount Rainier Exorcism, which will shock the lay reader as well as the most stringent demonologists, skeptics and scholars in the field of mental health.

I call this document, the Jesuit Report, the "da Vinci Code" of demonic possession and exorcism, since it reveals amazing mysterious information and events that will lead us to better understand the spiritual nature of man, as well as the events surrounding one of the most dramatic scenarios of the fight between good and evil. The body of a human being, through which the devil manifested his power contrary to God, became the peak manifestation of his opposition to Him and the control of the world. But let us not be so eager to rush to a spiritual conclusion based on the information contained in this Jesuit Report, since letters and interviews which may be on the contrary could hold the key to finally understanding the phenomena of demonic possession and exorcism via scientific means.

Finally, when I began writing this book, one of my colleagues at the Foundation for Research on the Nature of Man asked me, "Why another book on the case, with so many already written on the topic?" I responded that the issue remains important at the present time, not only because *The Exorcist* is still a scary movie, but also because the book and the film frame the long and ongoing religious and philosophical struggle between good, and evil and people from all walks of life are still interested in this subject. My effort also sheds new light on the investigation of this type of demonic possession cases from scientific, psychological, and religious perspectives, which will expand the knowledge about the case and clarify the truth behind the famous film with up-to-date dramatic information.

Introduction

As my sermon reached its climax in a local Mexican church in the summer of 1985, I began to feel uneasy with the way a young female adolescent, kneeling down before the altar, reacted anxiously to my words as I read from a biblical passage. I also noticed that some of the members of the prayer circle at my church were similarly reacting with uneasiness, as they closely observed her behavior. Suddenly, the 13-year-old girl stood up near the altar and began to speak in other tongues, or glossolalia (a phenomenon sometimes referred to as "ecstatic utterances," the uttering of unintelligible, language-like sounds while in a state of ecstasy), while performing grotesque body movements, accompanied by blasphemies against God, and squirting vomit towards the altar. These bizarre manifestations were interpreted by some of the church members as "sure signs that she was possessed by the devil."

The above case took place in my church shortly after the young lady had watched the movie *The Exorcist*, over ten years after the movie had been released in the early 1970s. This case is a reflection of the enormous impact the movie had on many people from different nations and cultures a long time after its release. The disturbing effects that the film could have on people, such as the young member of our church, to the point of causing her to feel that she was possessed by the devil, still remains intact even up to the present time. The psychological impact on this girl is an example of the influence of *The Exorcist*, which still reverberates many years later in some people.

In this book, the issues of exorcism and demonic possession and their meaning in the 21st century are extensively explored. Leading experts in the field of psychology, medicine, theology, and sociology face off on these controversial subjects. This book discusses the classical battle of science versus religion as well as good versus evil.

When writing his celebrated book, which he later adapted into the screenplay, William Peter Blatty certainly consulted experts and investigated demonic possession and exorcism in the context of which he completed his fictionalized story. However, he had in mind a particular case that had taken place, in Mount Rainier, Maryland, in 1949, and he had read about it in the *Washington Post* while he was a student at Georgetown University.

The newspaper report published by the *Washington Post* on August 20, 1949, was titled "Priest Frees Mount Rainier Boy Held in Devil's Grip," by Bill Brinkley. It became the main source for the story related by Blatty in his book. However, in order to protect the identity of the participants on the real case, Blatty changed the name of the 14-year-old male adolescent, as well as other participants in the Mount Rainier Exorcism. Most of the disturbing phenomena described in the novel and film also took place during the exorcism of the Mount Rainier adolescent, with the exception of the death of the exorcists.

There are many similarities and differences between *The Exorcist* and the Mount Rainier Exorcism, but the fact that such a dramatic novel and film were based on a true story leads us to wonder whether or not the incredible phenomena presented by Blatty in his book were accurate and truthful and could be validated. If so, the reports on the case would constitute one of the most powerful pieces of evidence in favor of the existence of the supernatural, and would shed a very powerful light on understanding more clearly the battle of science versus religion about the existence of the Devil and God in the universe. This is where the importance of the documents found, such as the Jesuit Report, lies; if truthful, it becomes a powerful smoking gun in favor of the existence of a spiritual world.

Such a complex endeavor as to prove or disprove the supernatural via the presentation of the information contained in the Jesuit Report constitutes a preposterous position for a scientific researcher on the Mount Rainier case. However, no one can deny that if the information is objective and truthful, and if after a careful scientific analysis of the case, we found that there is a high probability that the events as related in the Jesuit Report took place, we would have a firmer basis on which to rule out a natural or scientific explanation in favor of a supernatural one in the Mount Rainier Exorcism. This conclusion would point in the direction of confirming the existence of demonic possession and exorcism.

The book is outlined and organized with an initial account of the meaning of *The Exorcist* in the 21st century and how William Peter Blatty came across the story that inspired him to write the book and later the acclaimed film, followed by an account of the story of the Mount Rainier Exorcism. Next, complete detailed information on the events that surrounded the exorcism directly from the Jesuit Report is presented. Moreover, the information is framed on a scientific model proposed by John Nicola, author of the book *Diabolical Possession* and consultant to the film *The Exorcist* to evaluate it from a scientific standpoint.

The above model, which explores four dimensions of the investigation in cases of demonic possession and exorcism, is then applied to the actual case to determine its viability as an actual case of diabolical possession, rather than a case with a natural scientific explanation. Furthermore, principles of science are considered to determine if the case can be explained by fraud or by known scientific psychological or parapsychological mechanisms. As a scientist, I explore the case with the principle in mind that we do not have to recourse to supernatural explanations if natural explanations suffice, although they cannot be entirely denied nor disproved.

Also, in the context of the most rigorous scientific methodology, the real secrets behind *The Exorcist* and the causes of the paranormal phenomena surrounding it are examined. The information provided in this book will remove most the myths surrounding this famous case and will shock both believers and nonbelievers in exorcism and demonic possession. Moreover, in order to facilitate the reader's comprehension of the extensive material in the book, a section on questions that the reader may have in mind is included along with the responses.

Finally, to provide the reader with some of the most important sources on the book and the actual documents and interviews on the case, addendums are included of the correspondence between famous Duke University parapsychologist Dr. J.B. Rhine and the Rev. Luther Miles Schulze, the first minister to get in contact with the actual case. Secondly, the actual interviews are included with some of the witnesses of the Mount Rainier case who were still alive during my investigation. Also, fascinating interviews with international experts on demonic possession and religion are added, which address not only the case itself, but other complex related issues such as: whether the devil exists, the nature of evil, recollections from the first exorcism, and the sacred, the psychic and the scientific. Moreover, a section of illustrations are included of the actual places where the Mount Rainier Exorcism took place.

Although this book is written in a scholarly scientific style, still it addresses the issues in a simple language that can be understood not only by the scholarly reader, but also the lay person interested in learning about the true story behind *The Exorcist*.

1

In Search of Carl Jung's Mysterious Knife

Back in the summer of 1991, I was browsing in the archives of Foundation for Research on the Nature of Man (formerly the Duke Parapsychology Laboratory) at Duke University, looking for information on poltergeist phenomena for a paper that I had to complete for a course on anomalistic psychology at the Institute for Parapsychology in Durham, North Carolina. Suddenly, a thick bound book full of letters and correspondence from 1949, which I had been holding in my hand, fell onto the floor, face up. I leaned over and saw a letterhead featuring the name of a church, Saint Stephen's Evangelical Church. I picked the book up from the floor, curious about the church-related letter. As began to read, it stated, "We have in our congregation a family who are being disturbed by Poltergeist phenomena. They first appeared about January 15, 1949."

That letter caught my attention, as I vaguely recalled having read Denis Brian's biography of J.B. Rhine, *The Enchanted Voyager*, wherein he observed that the book titled *The Exorcist* had been based on an actual poltergeist case from 1949. As I continued to read the letter, I realized that the name of the reverend who wrote it was the same as that of the pastor in Brian's book. Later that day, I verified that it was, indeed, the same letter mentioned by Denis Brian in his book on the story of *The Exorcist*.

Finding the correspondence regarding the actual case on which William Peter Blatty based *The Exorcist* had been coincidental. Actually, as part of my academic assignment in psychology, I had been researching the archives looking for a story by Carl Jung relating the case of a knife that exploded inside a container while he was talking to a friend. However, that day I was excited instead by the letters that I had found by mere chance. Now that I had them, I was certain that they were related to the actual case on which *The Exorcist* was based.

At that point, memories came to me that, as an adolescent in the early seventies, I had watched the movie and had been shaken by the terrifying scenes of demonic possession that led me to develop fears of the Devil. Years later, as a member of the Pentecostal Church and a student of theology intending to become a minister of the church, I witnessed numerous cases that resembled the demonic or paranormal events presented in the famous book and the subsequent film. Indeed, the events of ostensible demonic possession that I witnessed had already aroused my interest in the topic, long before I undertook research on the real case behind *The Exorcist*.

Regarding the book and the film, I had always wondered if the story of *The Exorcist* was based on an actual event, as claimed by some newspapers suggesting that the real identities of the characters had been changed to protect their privacy. Later, during my years as a student of theology, I chose the topic of demonic possession and exorcism for the thesis I had to write for graduation. I was also wondering about the actual cases that occasionally took place in my church, where experiences of ostensible demonic possession appeared among some participants in the church's religious events and were treated spontaneously with prayers in the form of exorcism.

In contrast to other members of the church who were very eager to believe right away that these were actual cases of demonic possession, I took a very scientific approach and maintained an open mind. I had learned as a student of psychology to consider alternative natural hypotheses to explain the phenomena that I was witnessing. Unfortunately, my scientific curiosity was not welcomed by other members of the church, who considered that I was too skeptical and lacked faith. Nevertheless, I always defended my point that we needed to ascertain that these cases were genuine, so that we would not be deceived and be too eager to accept them as cases of genuine demonic possession. I was not a committed skeptic, but just had a critical mind and believed that, as a church, we would be better off adopting a more scientific attitude. At the same time, as a believer in the church dogma on demonic possession, I was certainly open to the idea that demonic possession could be the explanation when these cases simply could not be explained by a scientific hypothesis.

Over a period of more than 15 years, I had witnessed several dramatic cases of apparently possessed victims involved in some kind of paranormal phenomenon that resembled what Blatty had related in his dramatized story. In some cases, I saw other dramatic phenomena such as shaking mattresses, victims vomiting, physical contortions, apparent levitations, and even the death of the victim. Although I looked at these phenomena with a critical mind, some of the events were so impressive that it was hard for me to believe that the possessed victims were faking them. Then I began, along with a friend of mine who was a medical doctor, to investigate these cases in order to judge whether or not they were genuine examples of demonic possession.

If the evidence supported the church's hypothesis of demonic agency, I was prepared to uphold and confirm belief in the church dogmas. As it turned out, what I found was that church members tended to be overly careless and eager in assessing these cases, as they were reluctant to consider that they might not be genuine cases of demonic possession. In turn, this eagerness to believe in actual cases of demonic possession often led the church to hurt the "possessed victims" and their families, because instead of supporting them by violently ridding the possessed of their demons, we ended up alienating them and separating them from participation in church events and services.

In the early 1990s, I found myself again confronted with the topic of demonic possession and exorcism when I found the letters that were related to the actual case behind *The Exorcist* and the other text known as the Jesuit Report, which directly related the story behind the book. Both documents referenced the Mount Rainier Exorcism case on which Blatty had based most of his book. I decided, then and there, to research the case from a more scientific standpoint to search for the truth behind the story and determine whether or not the phenomena surrounding the case were real. I anticipated that this investigation would finally lead me to the confirmation of what I had previously believed, namely, that demonic possession existed and exorcism was the means to rid the possessed people of the demons and to cure them. This would corroborate my personal belief in the church doctrine on demonic possession that had been held for so many years. However, I also realized that I could use my research grant from the Parapsychology Foundation of New York, obtained with the purpose of investigating the actual exorcism case. In this way, I thought I could have the best of both worlds—that is, to confirm the church dogma on demonic possession and exorcism via a scientific methodology rather than simply as an acceptance of church doctrine.

That is why it was so exciting when I discovered the letters and the Jesuit Report on the Mount Rainier Exorcism, then decided to write a proposal for research funds to investigate the case. I was honored in 1992 to receive the first money ever granted by the Parapsychology Foundation of New York to study the Mount Rainier case. Moreover, the preliminary manuscript became the foundation of my doctoral dissertation, which was prepared under the guidance of the prestigious parapsychologists Stanley Krippner, Carlos Alvarado, and Nancy Zingrone, all of them former presidents of the Parapsychological Association.

In 1997, my research on the case came to the attention of Henninger Media Productions, a media company that was producing a scientific documentary for the Discovery Channel on the actual Mount Rainier case, based generally on Thomas Allen's book *Possessed*. I was then invited to participate in the documentary as an expert in the area of paranormal phenomena and psychology. Also, I had the honor to share in presenting the first scientific paper on the case at the 40th Scientific Congress of the Parapsychological Association held in Stockholm, Sweden, in 2006. It was the first time a paper on the topic of *The Exorcist* had been accepted by a refereed scientific committee to be given at a congress of this nature.

It is important to note, however, that my research is also based on personal interviews with people who participated in the Mount Rainier case and were still alive at the time the investigation was initiated. Among them were the Reverend Luther Miles Schulze, who granted me his first interview ever on the case, and his wife, then living at the Lutheran Retirement Home in Chevy Chase, Maryland. I also spoke with Ida Mae, who had been a member of the Circle of Prayers on behalf of the possessed adolescent in 1949 and was a close friend of the family; she also put me in touch with Ronald, the real possessed person in the Mount Rainier exorcism, with whom I was able to talk on the phone for almost half an hour.

For this book, the story also depended on the numerous exchanges of letters on the case between the famous parapsychologist J.B. Rhine and the Reverend Luther Miles Schulze—the ones I found by chance in the Duke Parapsychology Laboratory. Finally, I had the opportunity to access more data on the case, thanks to Anne Carroll, administrative and business manager of the Foundation of Research on the Nature of Man, who allowed me to search the organization's archives, where I found information on the actual Mount Rainier events in the Jesuit Report mentioned by Rhine in his correspondence on the case. It is on this document that I have relied for most of the details of the events that took place in the Mount Rainier Exorcism. It was Richard Broughton, Senior Research Scientist of the Foundation for Research, who gave me permission to use the correspondence between Rhine and Schulze and other related documents stored in the archives of the Foundation, an organization that owns the property rights of this very valuable collection of documents.

Of course, there are limitations of studying a case that took place more than sixty years ago. Since the Mount Rainier case took place so long ago, it is difficult to evaluate it, partially because the information I obtained in interviews may not be fully accurate, because of the time that has elapsed since the initial events took place. However, I am certain that, in spite of these limitations, this book provides key information that will remove some of the myths that surround both the Mount Rainier Exorcism and its subsequent dramatized version, *The Exorcist*.

Finally, *The Exorcist*, along with related writings and statements on the topics of possession and exorcism, has created a culture on diabolical possession and exorcism, leading people all over the world to continue to be interested in whatever is related to the fascinating story surrounding the book and the subsequent film. This book adds novel and fascinating information never previously published on the case. Even though more than sixty years have passed since the original case, and the fortieth anniversary of the film has been celebrated, the case still attracts the attention of readers and movie-goers, with the film often described as the most terrifying film in history. Therefore, any additional information on this fascinating case merits the attention of both believers in and doubters of demonic possession and exorcism.

2

The Exorcist Still Turns Heads in the Twenty-First Century

The possession case of Maria in my church resulted from a tsunami of terror and psychosis, inspired by the film *The Exorcist* back in the mid–70s among moviegoers and members of the church to which I belonged. It was a collective mental manifestation in which we began to see more cases of demonic possession than in recent memory. The case of Maria happened in the middle of this manifestation, which led many churchgoers to believe that she was really possessed by the Devil. At the time of this incident, I was a student of theology at the Pentecostal Biblical Institute Antioquia, where I was completing my studies to become a Pentecostal minister. The events actually happened during one of the sermons I was presenting at a local temple. Clearly, the film had not only impacted moviegoers, but also had an effect on members of my church.

Now we had a new concern in the church to worry about. Numerous cases of demonic possession seemed to be taking place shortly after the movie was released to the public in 1973, and even many years later. Were these the result of this collective mental manifestation caused by the impact of the film, or were they the result of a new manifestation of the Devil that we had ignored in the past? We realized that, for many years, the church had consigned cases of demonic possession and exorcism to the Middle Ages; it was obvious that we did not like to talk about or deal with these issues anymore. Certainly, *The Exorcist* brought a renewed attention to this topic in the early seventies, and now we had to deal with it.

At the present time, even in the twenty-first century, *The Exorcist* is still considered a seminal horror film in the history of moviemaking; it caused tidal waves of publicity and public reaction in the early 1970s, it continues to be effective today. For instance, in 1997, a documentary on *The Exorcist* and the actual story behind it was released by Henninger Media; according to some reports at the time, Warner Bros was planning a remake of the original film in 2007. Moreover, to some experts in filmmaking history, *The Exorcist* continues to be the most important horror movie of all time, even though the movie recently reached its 40th anniversary.

The reaction of terror evoked by the film in some of those who viewed it was so severe that, in some cases, psychiatric treatment was warranted. Moreover, what many people who watched the film initially ignored was that the book and later the acclaimed film were based on a real case that had taken place in the town of Mt. Rainier, Maryland, near Washington, D.C., in 1949.

The Exorcist is a distorted and exaggerated version of the aforementioned exorcism case. Over the years, this distorted version has been presented to the general public by the media as an accurate reflection of the true story. For instance, Father John L. Nicola in 1974, an expert on demonic possession who investigated the case, declared that the film reflected 90 percent of what actually happened.[1] Furthermore, the phenomenology of "supernatural nature" surrounding the fictionalized film, as well as the true story, have been portrayed in recent times by books such as Allen's *Possessed*, released in 1993, and documentaries such as *In the Grip of Evil*, produced by Henninger Media for the Discovery Channel in 1997. This film actually reflected to some extent most of the phenomenology surrounding the actual events behind *The Exorcist*.

Public Reaction to the Film

The movie frightened people in ways no other horror movie in history had done. Psychiatrists even coined the term "cinematic neurosis," for patients who left the movie feeling the presence of demons. The New Zealand Film Censor, for one, warned that parts of the film could be offensive or disturbing to some viewers.

Moreover, the reactions provoked by the horror movie not only affected millions of moviegoers, but also extended to well-educated groups such as theologians and psychiatrists, among whom an avalanche of reactions and comments were generated for and against the concepts of demonic possession and exorcism. Some of these reactions were published in refereed scientific journals and others in well-known popular and sensationalistic magazines. In this regard, Gunther in a special on *The Exorcist* for the *National Tattler*, a sensationalistic popular publication, in 1974[2] pointed out: "Like a volcanic eruption at the floor of a calm ocean, public reaction to the film, *The Exorcist*, has caused tidal waves of publicity unequaled in motion picture history. The gripping tale of a 12-year-old seized by an evil demon, *The Exorcist* either has been extolled or abhorred by religious leaders, medical authorities and people from every walk of life" (p. 4).

As hinted above, some of the reactions to the movie were so severe and adverse that psychiatric treatment was warranted for some viewers. For instance, William Taylor, a professor of psychology at the University of Wellington relates in a scientific journal[3] the cases of three moviegoers who required psychiatric intervention after viewing the film. Among them "is the case of a seventeen-year-old young man of high intelligence, with a long history of personality disorders that culminated in fainting fits, pyromania, and drug overdose, presented with visual and auditory hallucinations that were not unlike those he had watched in *The Exorcist*. He could not manage to sit all the way through the first performance, so he saw it again, to see if it would help him to see things more clearly. Instead, he continued to see people jumping on each other, and started when somebody inadvertently touched him. He awoke from a nightmare after the film as if possessed and took the place of a little girl" (p. 361).

Furthermore, the movie created a "collective psychosis" of supposed cases of demonic possession. Thus, similar cases in major religious groups were reported like never before in their history, to the point where religious authorities, Catholics as well as most Protestant denominations, had to take a stand regarding the topics of demonic possession and exorcism. Also, the movie, which some suspected at the time was based on a real case, was an embarrassment to the church, which in the 20th century had to take a public stand on the very controversial phenomena of demonic possession and exorcism. Indeed, the film brought a renewed attention to a topic that many psychiatrists and modern theologians had consigned to the Middle Ages and considered buried by our modern understanding of psychopathology.

Concerning the unusual interest and strong reaction provoked by the film, Taylor also stated: "The box office and extra-mural interest in possession and exorcism would suggest that writers of textbooks in psychopathology and psychiatry were premature in consigning those topics to brief historical sections relating to the pre-paradigmatic days of the development of science" (1975, p. 362).

More than 40 years have passed since *The Exorcist* was released as a novel and later as a movie; nevertheless, the reaction of terror created among lay people and in academic circles regarding the issue of possession continues to reverberate in the minds of many who viewed the film back in the '70s. In fact, it continues to spark interest even in the 21st century.

A Horror Film Born from a Newspaper Clipping

On August 20, 1949, the *Washington Post*[4] published an article by Bill Brinkley titled "Priest Frees Mount Rainier Boy Held in Devil's Grip." The newspaper related the story of a Catholic priest who had successfully exorcised the demon in an authentic Roman Catholic ritual from a 14-year-old boy who lived in Mount Rainier in Prince George's County, Maryland. The story read in part: "In what is perhaps one of the most remarkable experiences of its kind in church history, a 14-year-old Mount Rainier boy has been freed by a Catholic priest of possession by the Devil, Catholic sources reported yesterday. Only after 20–30 performances of the ancient ritual here and in St. Louis, was the Devil finally cast out of the boy" (p. 1A). The report on the case also indicated that the boy manifested violent tantrums and screaming, cursing and voicing of Latin phrases—a language he had never studied—whenever the priest read loudly the phrases of the Roman Ritual in which he commanded the demon to depart from the boy.

Nobody would have had ever imagined that, two decades later, the newspaper article on the Mount Rainier case would be used by William Peter Blatty, then a student at Georgetown University, who had become interested in the case after reading about it in the *Washington Post*, as the main possession case on which he would base his celebrated novel and later movie, *The Exorcist*. The fictionalized story deals with a 12-year-old girl who was possessed by the Devil after playing with a Ouija board.

3

The Exorcist and the 1949 Mount Rainier Exorcism Case

Certainly, William Peter Blatty drew from other historical cases of demonic possession and exorcism when writing his best-selling novel and later acclaimed film. Nevertheless, he had in mind a particular episode, the 1949 Mount Rainier case of a 14-year-old boy called Ronald, who apparently became possessed after experimenting with a Ouija board. However, in fictionalizing the Mount Rainier case in his novel, Blatty presented a 12-year-old girl instead of a boy in order to hide his identity. The girl, named Regan in the film, was played by Linda Blair. She was possessed by an evil spirit and performed incredible feats of body movement and physical strength. For example, she induced the levitation of objects in the room and, on occasions, squirted light green vomit toward people. In addition, marks appeared spontaneously on her body, and she was even able to turn her head completely backwards. She cursed people around her and, at one point, masturbated with a crucifix and then thrust her mother's face into her blood-filled crotch.

Blatty used most of the aforementioned physical feats and paranormal phenomena performed by the girl to embellish the original story, which was much less dramatic, and also to make it appear as a genuine case of demonic possession. It seems that he had read the Roman Ritual criteria for demonic possession and realized that, in order to meet the standards established by the Roman Ritual, he had to recreate the story to make it more appealing to moviegoers.

No doubt about it—the recreation of the real story was so impressive that it allowed him to achieve his goal of making it appear as a real case of demonic possession in both the novel and the film. Furthermore, the impact of terror caused by the dramatized film version on those who viewed it was tremendous, to the point where there were ambulances waiting outside some theaters in case someone watching the movie had medical or psychological reactions so severe as to require medical assistance.

However, what has Blatty himself said about the sources he used for the novel and film? Also, what were his intentions for writing *The Exorcist* in 1971? To what extent were the novel and the subsequent film based on the original Mount Rainier case? First of all, it is important to note that Blatty was not just writing a terrifying novel with fictional characters like most novels, but he was describing through the novel the reality of something that had happened. A report that appeared in the *Washingtonian* by Eddie Dean, titled "Think *The Exorcist* Was Just a Horror Movie? The Author Says You're Wrong," quotes William Peter Blatty: "Nobody's going to expect this to happen here," he says, "and that's what I was trying to get across: This is not a horror story. This is real. Something really happened here in Washington, D.C., with ordinary life buzzing all around" (October 2015).

Moreover, when writing his celebrated novel, which Blatty considered much more mysterious than the movie, he also had in mind a moral message to bring Americans back into church. In other words, he would use the movie to convey a moral message to a society in a nation that he considered to be in a moral crisis in the early seventies. In this regard, Nick Cull in an article published in *History Today* (May 2000) indicated: "*The Exorcist* was produced as a motion picture to scare a new generation of Americans back into church." Blatty was quite open about this aim. He called his novel "an apostolic work." He wanted to influence the society of his time by portraying incredible images of terror with a moral message embedded in them. It is important also to note that his novel and later film strengthened his Catholic faith, and as a writer he wanted to have a part in the church's message against the evil of the time.

Regarding his sources, he based most of the novel on the Mount Rainier Exorcism; he was able to contact the main exorcist of the case, and tried unsuccessfully to obtain a copy of the diary of the Mount Rainier Exorcism from the Catholic Church. However, he later declared that he had access to the diary after his novel was released. Had he had access to the complete story of the exorcism, perhaps the story of the film may have had much more complete details of the actual exorcism.

What were the reactions of experts on religion and mental health, as well as of the film industry? First, it is important to note that there were mixed reactions from those who were concerned about public morals. Many took exception to the depiction of blasphemous acts, child sexuality and the vivid representation of evil.

From the religious establishment, the reaction was adverse; the film was picketed by some clerics and condemned by the Protestant evangelist Billy

Graham. But the *Catholic News*, at least, suggested that the theme of evil was apposite for the age, and under the headline "Exorcist needs careful attention," urged viewers to look beyond the excesses of language and style.

At the present time, *The Exorcist* may be a sort of a joke for younger movie audiences, which is not surprising considering how many times it has been lampooned, even by Linda Blair herself in *Repossessed*. Yet, if they were to view the film in a more serious vein, not as just another creature feature, they may just find that there really is more to this film than a little girl spewing pea soup and spinning her head around 360 degrees. It is the ultimate battle between Heaven and Hell and Good and Evil. It is the story of the complete and total degradation of innocence. It is a study in character, and whether a man torn by the forces surrounding him can regain his faith in God and his belief in mankind to save the life of a little girl, caught up in forces beyond her control.

To what extent were the novel and the subsequent film based on the original Mount Rainier case? And can we consider the Mount Rainier case a "genuine" case of demonic possession, as Blatty makes it appear in his story? The question is important in the context of the analysis of the actual case, since it is believed, by some experts on demonology, that *The Exorcist* was based on a real and genuine case of demonic possession. Therefore, information that would shed light on the real case might finally clear up the myths that have surrounded *The Exorcist*.

Furthermore, *The Exorcist* brought a renewed attention to the topic of demonic possession; to some extent, it has served as a source or model of this type of case, in which the Church still believes, and which constitutes a dogma to which believers should adhere. Consequently, examination of *The Exorcist* and its source, the actual case, may shed light on the nature of these cases in order to determine whether they are real or fake. This is an important issue for believers who are sometimes eager to accept an account as genuine, based on their faith, without making a real scientific assessment of it.

Recent findings related to the case (Allen, 1993, and a further investigation by the author, Rueda, 1990–1993),[1] provide new information regarding the issue of whether or not Nicola was correct in his assessment of the Mount Rainier case. This new information suggests that Nicola's claims about how near the novel and the film were to the Mt. Rainier case were exaggerated. They clearly lack support from the new information provided from recent investigations of the case. Although there are some parallels between the film story and the real case, without the elements included by Blatty to dramatize the original story to make it appear as a real case of demonic possession, it would be very difficult to make a case in favor of a direct connection. Undoubtedly, Blatty exaggerated the original case in the fictionalized version to make it appear genuine, at least in terms of the standards established by the Ritual and the way some Catholic theologians defined it. The exaggerations helped the story fit the Catholic dogma of demonic possession and exorcism, a dogma as outlined by one of the most influential Catholic theologians and former official exorcist of the Vatican Corrado Balducci in his book *Diablo: ...Vivo e Atuante no Mundo* (1994).[2]

Ever since the film was released in the early 1970s, few details were known about the true story until very recently. Up to the present time, only partial information on the case had been leaked to the public, mostly through the popular press (Gunther et al., 1975). However, additional information was provided by Blatty himself in his subsequent book, *I'll Tell Them I Remember You* (1973).[3] Moreover, partial information on the case has been published in books and technical articles on parapsychology, such as Nicola's *Diabolical Possession and Exorcism* (1974) and Rogo's *The Poltergeist Experience* (1979).[4] Most of the known details regarding the true story behind *The Exorcist* come almost entirely from the partial information provided by the aforementioned sources and the film.

Ever since the Mount Rainier case took place, the Catholic Church has been reluctant to reveal any information about it, keeping the exorcism secret to protect the identity of the participants. Attempts to obtain the original church reports on the case were futile until recently, when new details about the Mount Rainier episode have come to light. A copy of a diary kept by one of the priests during the exorcism fell into the hands of Thomas Allen, a popular writer who presented *Possessed*, a more complete account of the case (1993). According to Allen, the diary, which mysteriously remained in a drawer of a table in a locked room at the Alexian Brothers Hospital in St. Louis, Missouri, was found by a worker when a construction company ordered that the building be torn down.

The diary used by Allen in his book, as well as his interviews conducted in 1991 and 1993 with some of the participants in and witnesses of the 1949 Mount Rainier Exorcism, provide us with a more complete picture. These sources delineate not only the true story behind Blatty's *The Exorcist*, but also furnish details of the psychological dynamics of the participants involved and the apparent paranormal phenomena they witnessed. This information, therefore, gives us a richness of elements with which to evaluate the Mount Rainier case from a psychological and parapsychological perspective in a more scientific context. However, Allen's account of the events, as presented in his book, is almost entirely a narrative of the case, with little attention provided to the more technical and scientific elements of it, even though the author tried to provide such an explanation at the end of the book. Unfortunately, as a writer of popular books, he lacked the training in mental health and illness to make his evaluation truly scientific.

The case was investigated by the famous parapsychologists J.B. Rhine and Louisa Rhine, from the Parapsychology Laboratory at Duke University, in 1949, when the actual events took place. They had learned about the case via lengthy correspondence with the Lutheran minister Luther Miles Schulze, to whom the parents of the "possessed" boy had appealed for help in the initial stages of the ordeal. It is important to note that, at this time, the case had not yet received the diagnosis of demonic possession by the Catholic Church. When the Rhines were invited by the Reverend Schulze to look into the case personally, they traveled to the Washington area to investigate it. Later, after having visited the premises and examined the place where the poltergeist-like phenomena had taken place, J.B. Rhine was quoted by a reporter from the *Washington Post* as having said that "it was the most impressive poltergeist phenomenon that had come to his attention" (Brian, 1982).[5] Concerning the 1949 Mount Rainier case, one of the exorcists in the case, Father William Bowdern, wrote to Blatty: "I can assure you of one thing: the case in which I was involved was the real thing [possession]. I had no doubt about it then and I have no doubt about it now."[6] Is Bowdern's assessment accurate? Was the 14-year-old boy Ronald really possessed by the Devil? Moreover, were the priests who determined that the case met the requirements of the Ritual for genuine cases of demonic possession accurate in their assessment? Or, on the contrary, was it instead a psychiatric problem or poltergeist case masked by religious beliefs? Furthermore, would deliberate fraud be a viable explanation in the case? Or were the exorcists genuinely convinced of the need for their ministrations? Some of these questions have been in the minds of millions of moviegoers and experts, who read the novel and viewed the film *The Exorcist*, since it was released in 1973. Among them are psychologists, psychiatrists, religious authorities, and other experts in the fields of psychology and theology, who have expressed their reservations in the case.

I will attempt to review and answer some of the above questions in the context of what it is known and has been published on the Mount Rainier case ever since the early 1970s, particularly in terms of information that has come to light more recently. I will focus on analyzing the case in the context of viable hypotheses that may explain the phenomena in terms of what is known in science, without discarding its paranormal and religious aspects. First, I will summarize the case itself, based on information from various published sources, and will attempt to reconstruct the events as they took place. These sources now include some recent interviews with witnesses who are still alive, who participated in events of the 1949 Mount Rainier case. This summary of the case story will not be exhaustive. It will stress the most salient aspects of the case as well as highlight the parapsychological phenomena that surrounded it; these can help us assess the case and the events in the light of what science has to say about these types of phenomena.

Secondly, I will evaluate the case from four different angles and hypotheses—fraud, psychology, poltergeists, and the theory of diabolical agency. I will also, when evaluating the evidence of the case, have in mind some principles of science and sound principles to investigate demonic possession proposed by science and some Christian theologians:

- The Laplace Principle: States that "we should not reject phenomena we cannot explain" but that "we must examine them with an attention all the more scrupulous as they seem more difficult to admit."[7]
- Scientific economy: "If a natural hypothesis can explain the phenomena we do not have to have recourse to a supernatural causal agency to explain a paranormal or supernatural phenomenon." In other words, as stated by theologian Juan Cortes, "A supernatural explanation of the facts may be accepted only when every natural explanation is incapable of doing so."[8]
- Science Cannot Provide Complete Answers to All Questions: There are many matters that cannot usefully be examined in a scientific way. There are, for instance, beliefs that—by their very nature—cannot be proved or disproved (such as the existence of supernatural powers and beings, or the true purposes of life). In other cases, a scientific approach that may be valid is likely to be rejected as irrelevant by people who hold to certain beliefs (such as in miracles, fortune-telling, astrology, and superstition). Nor do scientists have the means to settle issues concerning good and evil, although they can sometimes contribute to the discussion of such issues by identifying the likely consequences of actions, which may be helpful in weighing alternatives.

Although the Laplace principle does not refer precisely to a phenomenon of supernatural nature, I will use the principle loosely to refer to the fact that we must examine a hypothesis with the utmost attention, particularly if it is difficult to admit, such as the existence of demonic possession, since this is a causal hypothesis difficult to admit in terms of what we know about science. In reference to the principle of scientific economy, we will not have recourse to a supernatural agency to explain phenomena that may be explained by natural means. For instance, in the Mount Rainier case, there is a phenomenon of branding and marks that appeared on the adolescent that may be explained by a normal dermatological mechanism.

It is important to note that, even though I cite the above principles and suggestions as guidance in evaluating the Mount Rainier case, I do not want to make the reader think that such complex issues like demonic possession are necessarily subject to the above principles. As previously indicated, the evidence we are examining in the context of four hypotheses comes from anecdotal evidence, the stories of ordinary witnesses about paranormal of supernatural events.

This evidence is usually uncritical and has the tendency to become embroidered with the passing of time. Consequently, I will try to frame the information on the case and the hypothesis examined in the context of the above suggested principles.

4

Overview of the 1949 Mount Rainier Exorcism

The Visit from Top Researchers of the Paranormal: A Poltergeist Case?

The news about the Mount Rainier case reached J.B. Rhine and Louisa Rhine, famous parapsychologists from the Duke University Parapsychology Laboratory, through the Lutheran minister Luther Miles Schulze, to whom the family of the apparently possessed 14-year-old boy had appealed for help. In a letter addressed to J.B. Rhine, director of the institute, on March 21, 1949, Schulze stated:

> We have in our congregation a family who are being disturbed by poltergeist phenomena. It first appeared about January 15, 1949. The family consists of the maternal grandmother, a fourteen-year-old boy, who is an only child, and his parents. The phenomenon is apparent only in the boy's presence. I had him in my home on the night of February 17–18 to observe by myself. Chairs moved with him and one threw him out. His bed shook whenever he was in it. When he was in bed with me, mine vibrated. There was no apparent motion of his body. I then made a bed on the floor for him and this glided over the floor.... Would you or someone from your staff be interested in studying this case? The family mentioned other such phenomena as chairs moving, tables over-turning, and objects flying, and scratching and drumming. Their floors are scarred from the sliding of heavy furniture.[1]

Details of the phenomena surrounding the boy, as described by Schulze, prompted the interest of the Rhines in the case, some parts of which seemed to them to be of a possible poltergeist nature. However, they could provide a neutral analysis in the context of which they explained that the adolescent himself may have been responsible for causing the phenomena. As for Schulze's request for help, Rhine responded that he was deeply interested in

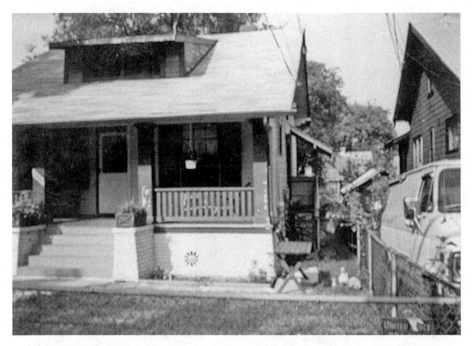

This is one of the houses where the Hunkeler family lived during part of the ordeal of Ronald's exorcism, located in Rockville, Maryland, at 3807 40th Drive, Cottage City, Maryland (1993).

the case, that he was going through Washington several times that spring, and that he would stop off in the area if he knew he could be of any help.

In the meantime, he offered Schulze a preliminary explanation of the possible causes of the phenomena described in his letter. In his reply, he wrote: "As you know, the most likely normal explanation is that the boy is, himself, led to create the effect of being the victim of mysterious agencies or forces and he might be sincerely convinced of it. Such movements as those of the chair and the bed might, from your very brief account of them, have originated within him. Presumably, however, the movement of the bed on the floor was not of that type. I presume you observed the movement in good light and were not relying on his account of it."[2] The psychokinetic phenomena such as chairs that moved, as related by Schulze to Dr. Rhine in this letter, sounded to him like those phenomena present in some classical poltergeist cases.

Later, when the Rhines personally traveled to Washington to investigate the case, they examined the minister's room, where Ronald had spent the night with the Reverend Schulze, who witnessed the phenomena that he was unable to explain. According to Schulze's letter to Dr. J.B. Rhine, the initial

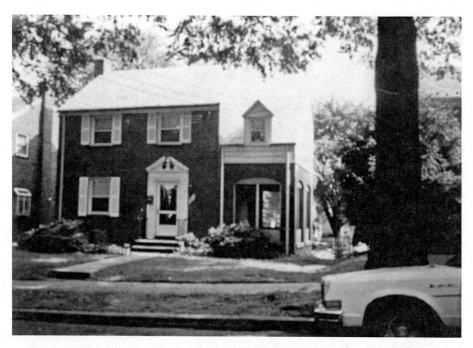

This is the house where the Reverend Luther Schulze lived, located at 1647 Varnum Place N.E., Washington, D.C. Ronald spent the night here with the Reverend Schulze, who witnessed some of the most amazing phenomena (1993).

manifestations that he witnessed of the case that took in his house, located at 1647 Varnum Place N.E., Washington, D.C.

Communication from the Dead: The Deceased Aunt

According to the story related in the Jesuit Report[3] sent to Dr. J.B. Rhine, the manifestation of the strange phenomena began on January 15, 1949. Ronald and his grandmother were at home by themselves when the supernatural presence was first felt. As described in the Jesuit Report:

> On January 15, 1949, at the home of XXXXXXXX in Cottage City, Maryland a dripping noise was heard by XXXXXXX and his grandmother in the grandmother's bedroom. This noise was continued for a short time and then the picture of Christ on the wall shook as if the wall back of it had been bumped. By the time the parents of R returned home there was a very definite scratching sound under the floor boards near the grandmother's bed. From this night on, the scratching was heard every night about seven o' clock and would continue until midnight. The family thought that the scratching was caused by rodent of some kind. An exterminator was called

in who placed chemicals under the floor boards, but the scratching sound continued and became more distinct when people stamped on the floor (J.R., p. 1).

The scratching noise continued for another ten days before it stopped.

Three days later, another sound was heard, this time in Ronald's bedroom on the first floor. While Ronald, his mother, and his grandmother were lying on the bed, they heard something sounding like squeaky shoes, apparently coming towards them, similar to the rhythm of marching feet and the beat of drums.

The sounds continued repeatedly until Ronald's mother asked: "Is that you, Aunt Dorothy"?[4] (p. 1, J.R.). It is important to note the role that Aunt Dorothy played in the case. She was Ronald's recently deceased aunt, who used to live in St. Louis, Missouri, and had an avid interest in spiritualist practices. Also, as a frequent visitor to the family, she had developed a special relationship with Ronald, having introduced him to the Ouija board and other spiritualist devices, which she used to contact the other world. Concerning Aunt Dorothy's interests in spiritualist practices, Thomas Allen, the author of the book *Possessed*, regarding this case (1993)[5] observed:

[She] ... was a Spiritualist; she saw it to make contact between this world and the next. The planchette, she explained to [Ronald], would sometimes move in response to answers given by the spirits of the dead (pp. 2, 3).
    Aunt Harriet told Robbie and Phyllis that, lacking a Ouija board, spirits could try to get through this world by rapping on walls (p. 3).

Note: Allen uses the names Robbie for Ronald and Phyllis for Dorothy.

Moreover, according to Allen, Aunt Dorothy's teachings on spiritualism and her practice with the Ouija board would influence Ronald later to make use of that board to try to reach his deceased aunt. Furthermore, this may also explain why Ronald's mother, influenced by the teachings of her sister-in-law on how spirits communicate with this world through rapping on the walls, would suspect that Aunt Dorothy was trying to communicate with them through that means.

Another incident that might have influenced Ronald's family to imagine a connection between the strange sounds happening at home and the death of Aunt Dorothy was a series of unexplained phenomena that had occurred when the family took a Sunday ride with her. First, a lap robe in the back seat of the car began to curl up. Later, an invisible force pushed Ronald and his mother against the seat. Finally, when they returned to Aunt Dorothy's home, Ronald's father reached for the ignition to shut off the engine, but the key was not in the switch. He later discovered it under the front seat, where it had apparently lain for much of the drive.

The incidents may well have led the family to believe that there was a connection between the strange sounds and Ronald's aunt. Therefore, to find out if Aunt Dorothy was behind the phenomena manifested, Ronald's mother organized a séance. During this séance, when a phenomenon would occur, the mother asked: "Is this you, Aunt Dorothy?" But there was no answers. "If you are Dorothy," said the mother again, "knock three times." Waves of air struck the grandmother, mother, and boy in the face; then three distinct knocks were heard on the floor. The mother said, "If you are really Dorothy, knock four times." Claw scratching on the mattress followed the four raps" (p. 1, J.R.).

"When the mother or grandmother paid no attention to the mattress scratching, the entire mattress would begin to shake. On one occasion, the coverlet was pulled out from the mattress with its edges standing up above the surface of the bed in a curled form as though held up with starch. When a bystander touched the bedspread, the sides fell back into a normal position. The scratching on the mattress was continuous since the first night it was heard" (p. 3, J.R.).

The Circle of Prayers

The Reverend Schulze then asked the family to let Ronald stay at his home overnight, so that he himself could see the phenomena surrounding

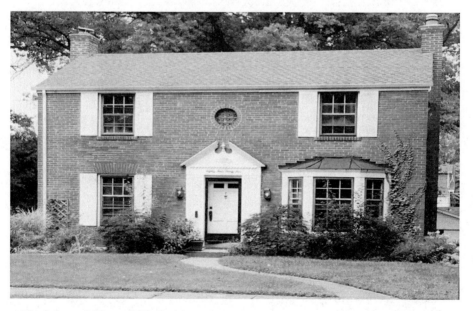

The house of the Hunkeler family in St. Louis, Missouri, where most of the strange phenomena took place (1993).

the boy. Since the manifestations persisted at Schulze's home, he called on another minister to assist him. Together they tried to help the family by organizing circles of prayer at the church and at the family's home. One of the participants in these circles, Ida Mae, whom I interviewed personally, was a very active member of Schulze's congregation and a close friend of Ronald's family. She related that during one of the prayer circles organized at the family's house, she witnessed an apparent levitation of Ronald from the bed. As she recalled:

> The boy was lying on the bed when we initiated the prayers. He suddenly broke into screaming and cursing those around him. He appeared to be speaking in a language other than English; the sounds and the words did not resemble those of the English language. Somebody present in the room commented later that he was probably speaking in Latin. As he cursed those around him who were reading the Bible, I was standing in front of him and noticed that his body, lying flat on the bed, began to rise slowly from it. His body seemed to be completely separate from the bed about two inches and then fell back.[6]

The First Formal Report of the Mount Rainier Case

In the next sequence of events, we have outlined the story as related to Rhine Schulze, who prepared a report of these events, which was sent along with the famous Jesuit Report. In the report, this section is titled "Case report or background information for the case." This report is also mentioned initially in the correspondence between the Reverend Schulze and Dr. J.B. Rhine. In a letter addressed to the Reverend Schulze, Dr. Rhine stated, "We are very much indebted to you for the trouble to which you have gone in preparing the report of the Ronald case. Dick Darnell just sent me a copy." Also, the following events are also based on the personal interviews that were conducted with the Revered Luther Schulze.

The Skeptical Minister: The Shocking Phenomena at His Premises

Regarding the night that Ronald spent at Schulze's home, the minister related that Ronald's father brought him over after dinner and then left. Schulze reassured the boy, "You are going to have a good night's sleep." Then he let him take his own bed. (The minister and his wife had twin beds; his wife had agreed to spend that night in a guest room adjoining the master bedroom.) Schulze decided to leave the room clearly lit throughout the night, saying to himself, "Nothing ever happens here." Then they both said their prayers and wished each other a good night. Sometime later, Schulze heard Ronald's bed creaking; putting out his hand, he touched the boy's bed and felt it shaking, "like one of those motel vibrator beds, but much faster." As he recalled, "Ronald was still awake, but there was no apparent motion of his body while the bed was moving."

Next, the Reverend Schulze asked the boy to get out of the bed and rest in a heavy chair, one with a very low center of gravity. Soon after the boy sat down there, the minister reported, "I saw the chair start moving; it went backwards several inches and turned over with the boy on it." As Schulze recalled, it moved against the wall as far as it would go. Then it turned around and tipped over, with the boy still sitting on the chair. The Reverend Schulze estimated that the chair took more than a minute to land on its side and deposit Ronald almost gently on the floor. According to the Reverend Schulze, while the chair moved, Ronald appeared to be in some kind of trance. After the boy was tipped out of the chair, the minister suggested that the floor was the safest place for him to rest. He recalled, "Then I asked Ronald to lie on the floor on the scatter rug, and I arranged a goatskin for a mattress and a blanket to cover him, at the foot of one of the beds. Then I retired to my bed."

Soon after, he observed, "I saw Ronald and the bed moving as a unit across the floor. Under one of the beds, Ronald's hands were visible. I could also see his legs outlined. They were stretched out and still, which rules out normal propulsion with hands and feet; the blankets were not even wrinkled." After witnessing these phenomena, Schulze realized he was witnessing something that he could not explain. As he recalled, "Something strange was happening there ... the boy was not faking it.... I wondered if I was going screwy."

The Reverend Schulze's home was not a haven from the strange phenomena that had manifested in the boy's own home. Because of the experience, he tried to persuade Ronald's parents to have him examined by a doctor. As he noted, "I wanted to put him in the hands of our family doctor, who I knew was going to be sympathetic to the case, but his parents would not let me do it." Neither could their family doctor get consent to put him in a hospital. Instead of following Schulze's advice to have Ronald examined by a doctor, they decided to call a spiritualist to see if that person could free Ronald.[7]

The Confrontation: A Skeptical Reverend Defies a Spiritualist

The family did, indeed, call in a spiritualist to help him. As Schulze recalled, this was a woman who did spirit anointing in order to rid people of spirits. She saw the boy at a time when the minister was there as well. He noted, "She was trying to prove to us that she had powers, and performed some magic tricks that I was able to replicate. I remember now that this woman folded a piece of paper and then it opened up. I did the same thing with a piece of paper, and it would open for anybody. I said, 'Look! I can do the same thing,' and she thought I had stolen some of her thunder."

According to the Reverend Schulze, the family's attempt to aid Ronald through a spiritualist failed. Ronald's condition remained unchanged. Finally, Schulze was able to persuade the family to have Ronald examined by a physician. The boy was placed in the hands of the county's mental hygiene clinic, under Dr. Mabel Ross of the University of Maryland. She and her staff had two interviews with him. Meanwhile, the family's personal physician persisted in treating the boy with an anti-epileptic medication called Barbital.

In addition, Father Albert Hughes of St. James Catholic Parish in Mount Rainier was also consulted; he suggested the use of blessing candles, holy water, and special prayers to rid the boy from the forces that were affecting him. His mother followed his advice and started using these procedures at

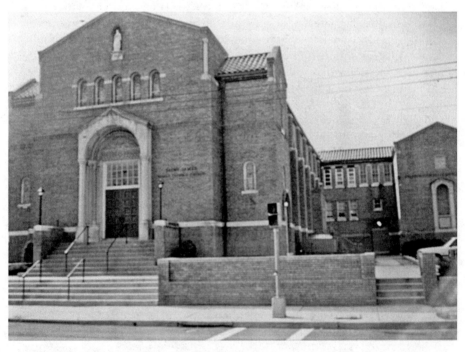

St. James Catholic Church, where the Hunkelers were sent by the Reverend Schulze to seek out help for their son. Schulze told them about the exorcism ritual practiced by Catholic priests, whom he said may be of help to Ronald. The church later became, according to Ida Mae, a Baptist church (1993).

home, but the situation did not change much, nor did the condition of the adolescent improve. The phenomena surrounding Ronald continued to take place, despite the rituals performed by the family, as the mother reported.

For instance, on one occasion, the mother took a bottle of holy water and sprinkled it around all the rooms. After finishing, she placed the bottle on a dresser; it then seemed to be picked up by something and smashed. Once, when she lit the candles, three flames soared to the ceiling.

Poltergeist–like Phenomena at Home and School

The strange phenomena taking place around Ronald even seemed to follow him to school. For example, on one occasion, when he was at school, his desk moved around on the schoolroom floor. Because of the bizarre events that continued to take place around Ronald, his parents decided to stop sending him to school. As related in the Jesuit Report:

> An orange and a pear flew across the entire room where R. was standing. The kitchen table was upset without any movement on the part of R. Milk and food were thrown off the table and stove. The breadboard was thrown on to the floor. Outside the kitchen a coat on its hanger flew across the room; a comb flew violently through the air and extinguished blessed candles; a Bible was thrown directly at the feet of R., but did not injure him in any way. While the family was visiting a friend in Boonesborough, Maryland, the rocker in which R. was seated spun completely around through no effort on the part of the boy. R's desk at school moved about on the floor similar to the plate on a Ouija board. Therefore, Ronald did not continue his attendance of school out of embarrassment (p. 2, J.R.).

5

Demonic Possession

Some Concepts and the First Exorcism of Ronald

As the strange phenomena continued to happen around the boy, the family somehow began to believe God was punishing them for leaving the Catholic Church, since they had converted to the Lutheran Church. Therefore, they decided to consult a Catholic priest, Father Albert Hughes, from St. James Catholic Church, who agreed to visit Ronald and talk to him.

According to one version, the initial phenomenon that he witnessed was Ronald speaking Latin, a phenomenon designated as xenoglossy (the putative paranormal phenomenon by which a person can speak or write a language he or she could not have acquired by natural means). Another version of the case indicates that a rabbi, whom the family had also called in to examine Ronald, heard him speaking Hebrew. When a professor of Oriental languages was also invited to come by, he voiced the opinion that Ronald was speaking Aramaic.

"After having examined Ronald for some time, Father Hughes considered that he had heard enough and that the boy presented the symptoms of demonic possession. He, then, decided to request permission from the Archbishop to perform an exorcism on Ronald" (p. 3, J.R.), at Georgetown Hospital. When permission was granted, he prepared himself for the exorcism. However, before moving on to the details of the exorcism of Ronald, it is important that we become familiar with the signs that Father Hughes may have observed that led him to conclude that Ronald was possessed and that he required an exorcism to free him from the demon. Below is a brief description of demonic possession, exorcism and related concepts, according to Catholic beliefs, to help the reader reach a better understanding of the phenomena surrounding Ronald and the reason for the priest's decision to perform the ritual exorcism.

What Is Demonic Possession?

According to Oesterreich,[1] an expert in demonic possession, it "is as if another soul had entered into the body and henceforward subsisted there, in place of or side by side with the normal subject, in this case, the demon is the one who enters the body of the possessed individual" (p. 17). According to Father Gabriel Amorth, the prestigious official exorcist of the Vatican, in his book *An Exorcist Tells His Story*,[2] demonic possession occurs when Satan takes full possession of the body (not the soul); he speaks and acts without the knowledge or consent of the victim, who therefore is morally blameless. It is the gravest and most spectacular form of demonic afflictions.

Moreover, it is important to note that in many cultures and in many belief systems, particularly in Christianity, it is believed that the spirit possession of an individual is caused by a malevolent preternatural being, commonly known as a demon. Among some of the signs of demonic, according to father Amorth[3] and other experts in demonic possession, we have:

Transformation of the physiognomy or physical appearance of the possessed.
Speaking in tongues or foreign languages (xenoglossy).
Erased memories or personalities of the possessed.
Convulsions, "fits" and fainting as if one were dying.
Access to hidden knowledge (gnosis).
Drastic changes in vocal intonation and facial structure.
The sudden appearance of injuries (scratches, bite marks) or lesions
Extraordinary or superhuman strength.

Unlike channeling, the subject has no control over the possessing entity, so it will persist until forced to leave the victim, usually through a form of exorcism.

What Is Exorcism?

On the other hand, exorcism (from the Greek ἐξορκισμός, exorkismos— binding by oath) is defined by *The Catholic Encyclopedia*[4] as (1) the act of driving out, or warding off, demons or evil spirits from persons, places, or things, which are believed to be possessed or infested by them, or are liable to become victims or instruments of their malice; (2) the means employed for this purpose, especially the solemn and authoritative adjuration of the demon in the name of God, or any other higher power to which he is subject. Depending on the spiritual beliefs of the exorcist, this may be done by causing the entity to swear an oath, by performing an elaborate ritual, or simply by commanding it to depart in the name of a higher power. The practice is ancient and part of the belief system of many cultures and religions.

In the case of Ronald, since he was in the hands of a Catholic priest, the exorcism to be performed was based on a particular format or procedures contained in the famous Roman Ritual (in Latin, Rituale Romanum).

What Is the Roman Ritual?[5]

It is one of the official ritual works of the Roman Rite of the Catholic Church. It contains all of the services that may be carried out by a priest or deacon on those diagnosed as being possessed by the Devil, as determined by the signs listed in the Roman Ritual.

The Failed Initial Exorcism

The next sequence of events led to the first and second exorcisms of Ronald that took place shortly after the participation of the Rev. Luther Schulze in the case. The story is based on the Jesuit Report that the Rev. Luther Miles Schulze obtained from Ronald's family (who in turn obtained it from the priests who conducted the second exorcism of the adolescent). The Jesuit Report, quite an extensive document, was sent to Dr. J.B. Rhine for his evaluation by the Rev. Luther Miles Schulze. This document was obtained from the personal correspondence of Dr. Rhine and Louisa Rhine, housed at the Foundation for Research on the Nature of Man, located in Durham, North Carolina. I also obtained a copy from Ida Mae, the personal assistant to the Reverend Schulze back in the 1940s.

Most of the archives of the former Institute of Parapsychology at Duke University became part of Duke's Perkins Library. However, a lot of the personal correspondence did not become part of the collection at Perkins Library, and remained at the Foundation for Research on the Nature of Man. With the help of Anne Carrol, business manager and personal secretary of Dr. J.B. Rhine for over 30 years, the Jesuit Report and other relevant information was found. Permission was granted to the author by Anne Carrol and Richard Broughton (director of research at the Foundation) to use it for his investigation of the Mount Rainier Exorcism. I will next summarize the most salient events related to the main exorcism of Ronald, based on the Jesuit Report.

The following sequence of events reveals what happened during the first exorcism performed on Ronald, one that initially failed but later was resumed by the Jesuit priests at the Alexian Brothers Hospital in St. Louis. Moreover,

Father Albert Hughes, now in charge of the Mount Rainier case, was convinced that this was an actual case of demonic possession, and prepared accordingly to perform the exorcism on Ronald. He took time for fasting and prayers. According to the Catholic Church Ritual of Exorcism, the following preparations and procedures are essential:

The priest delegated by the Ordinary to perform this office should first go to confession or at least elicit an act of contrition, and, if convenient, offer the holy Sacrifice of the Mass, and implore God's help in other fervent prayers. He vests in a surplice and a purple stole. Having before him the person possessed (who should be bound if there is any danger), he traces the sign of the cross over him, over himself, and over the bystanders, and then sprinkles all of them with holy water. After this he kneels and says the Litany of the Saints, exclusive of the prayers which follow it. All present are to make the responses (p. 1).

The Litany of the Saints is used in ordination, Forty Hours, processions, and other occasions. Both the Roman Ritual and the Roman Pontifical direct that the first three invocations be repeated. The music for this litany is given in the music supplement. The invocations are sung (or recited) by the chanters or the priest, the responses by all.

P: Lord, have mercy.
ALL: Lord, have mercy.
P: Christ, have mercy.
ALL: Christ, have mercy.
P: Lord, have mercy.
ALL: Lord, have mercy.
P: Christ, hear us.
ALL: Christ, graciously hear us.

The above prayers must have been part of the Litany of the Saints with which Father Hughes initiated the exorcism.

Therefore, in accordance with the prescribed procedures, once Father Hughes arrived at the place where the exorcism was going to be conducted, he had to make sure that the boy did not hurt himself during the ordeal and that he, the priest, had control of the situation. The first thing he did before initiating the exorcism was to order straps to be attached to the bed to hold Ronald during the ritual. Soon after that, he initiated the exorcism according to the instructions of the Roman Ritual, beginning with reciting the preliminary prayers as directed. As he continued reciting the prayers, Ronald somehow managed to move one of his arms under the straps; he was able to slide his hand out of the bed, whereupon he grabbed a loose piece of the bedsprings and slashed Hughes's arm from shoulder to wrist. The wounds caused by the slash required one hundred stitches to close. After this incident, Father Hughes decided to cease the exorcism and disappeared from the scene. This sequence of events is reminiscent of the one in the movie *The Exorcist*, in which one of the priests is psychologically attacked by the demon possessing Linda Blair and is then asked by the main exorcist to leave the room; however, father Damian Karras stays during the entire exorcism assisting Father Lankester Merrin. In the particular case of the Mount Rainier Exorcism, this first attempt to rid the Ronald from the possessing entity ended in a dramatic way when Father Hughes was injured very severely. It is very likely that as a result of this very severe injury of the shoulder and arm, the medical consequences may have been serious, and the injury may have left a permanent scar on the body of the exorcist. After this failed exorcism, the family consulted Fathers William Bowdern and Frank Bishop, who decided to take the adolescent to St. Louis to the Alexian Brothers Hospital, where a second exorcism took place.

The Second Exorcism: The Deliverance from Evil

After Ronald and his family arrived in St. Louis, the events that took place now led to the second exorcism of Ronald, performed by Catholic priests William Bowdern and Frank Bishop. One of them carefully began a report of the events as they took place, prior to and after the exorcism performed on the adolescent, including the previous events observed by family members and other witnesses. The priest who reported the events started with an introduction of a "Case Study," which constitutes a very complete and detailed account of the events surrounding the Mount Rainier Exorcism. It also includes a detailed account of what happened during the second exorcism, throughout the entire procedure, until after the adolescent was freed via the exorcism. It starts with a title: "Report of events of the Exorcism of Ronald"; secondly, sketchy biographical information of Ronald is included. To facilitate the reader's grasp of the sequence of events of the second exorcism, between dated historical accounts of the case, I will start each dated section with a subtitled and brief introduction, which is not part of the original document. Also, where there are similarities to the movie *The Exorcist*, I will indicate it as complementary information for the reader.

6

The Jesuit Report
The Exorcism of Ronald

Note: The Jesuit Report is reproduced as it was found originally, unedited.

Background Information
March 7, 1949
Birth: 1935
Religion: Evangelical Lutheran, baptized 6 mo. after birth by a Lutheran Minister
Maternal Grandmother: Practicing Catholic until the age of 14
Paternal Grandfather: Baptized Catholic but no practice
Father: Baptized Catholic but no instruction or practice
Mother: Baptized Lutheran
Ronald and his mother visited St. Louis at the home of Mr. and Mrs. XXXXX

The Jesuit Document, after presenting the initial biographical information of Ronald and his family, next presents a section called Case Study, where the Jesuit Priest who wrote this document begins with an account of the strange events that led the family to seek help with their minister. In the next chapter, the report presents the events surrounding the Mount Rainier Exorcism in a very detailed sequence. However, a summary will be presented next of the main events surrounding it, including quotations about the information of the exorcism as it appears in the original document.

Note: In the report Xs were used to provide privacy, *s indicate illegibility of text, and incomplete or incoherent excerpts suggest that profane text had been marked out on the original.

Also, it is important to note that in this Jesuit Report, the name of Ronald appears with a single R, when the report refers to him. Finally, at the end of each section of the Jesuit Document cited, I use the letters J.R., to refer to the Jesuit Report along with the corresponding page where the text cited comes from. Also, thematic subheads are used to facilitate the reading of very long descriptions of the events as related by the report.

How It All Began

January 15, 1949

On January 15, 1949, at the home of XXXXXXXX in Cottage City, Maryland a dripping noise was heard by XXXXXXX and his grandmother in the grandmother's bedroom. This noise was continued for a short time and then the picture of Christ on the wall shook as if the wall back of it had been bumped. By the time the parents of R returned home there was a very definite scratching sound under the floorboards near the grandmother's bed. From this night on, the scratching was heard every night about seven o'clock and would continue until midnight. The family thought that the scratching was caused by a rodent of some kind. An exterminator was called in who placed chemicals under the floorboards, but the scratching sound continued and became more distinct when people stamped on the floor.

This scratching continued for ten days and then stopped. The family finally believed that the rodent had died. The boy, R, seemed to think he still heard the noise but the family did not hear anything for a period of three days. When the sound became audible again, it was no longer in the upstairs bedroom but had moved downstairs in the boy's bedroom. It was heard as the sound of squeaking shoes along the bed and was heard at night only when the boy went to bed. The squeaking sound continued for six nights, and on the sixth night scratching again was audible. The mother, grandmother and boy while lying on the bed on this night heard something coming toward them similar to the rhythm of marching feet and the beat of drums (p. 1, J.R.).

Six weeks later, after the first mysterious sound was heard at Ronald's house, blood-red marks emerged on Ronald's skin reading "Louis." Ronald's mother, who looked at the marks, assumed that they were an indication that they had to take him to that city. Next, when they wondered when they should leave, the word Saturday appeared as a red mark on his skin. As to the length of time the mother and the boy should stay in St. Louis, another mark was printed on the boy's chest, this one reading "3½ weeks," answering possible questions on the destination departure, and duration of the trip. The Jesuit Document relates the event as follows:

> On one evening the word "Louis" was written on the boy's ribs in deep red. Next when there was some question of the time of departure, the word "Saturday" was written plainly on the boy's hip. As to the length of time the mother and boy should stay in St. Louis, another message was printed on the boy's chest, "3½ weeks." The printing always appeared without any motion on the part of the boy's hands. The mother was keeping him under close supervision (p. 2, J.R.).

In the film *The Exorcist*, even though no such complicated series and sequential scratches or marks appeared on the possessed adolescent, letters did appear on her body in the form of the word HELP; these were witnessed by Father Karras, the young Catholic priest initially involved in the case, as he continued his search of evidence in order to determine if this was an actual case of demonic possession. In Ronald's case, the family, compelled by the messages on his body, decided to take him to St. Louis, where they had relatives. They stayed in the home of the boy's non–Catholic aunt and uncle.

Next, new marks appeared to others who were questioning whether Ronald should be sent to school while in St. Louis. The Jesuit Report relates: "There seemed to be a sharp pain when the marks occurred so that the boy doubled up and uttered a rather terrifying sound. The markings could not have been done by the boy for the added reason that on one occasion there was writing on his back. Even in St. Louis the writing continued. There was some question of sending R. to school during his visit here, but the message, 'No,' appeared on his wrists; also a large 'n' on both legs. The mother feared disobeying this order."

Furthermore, the Jesuit who wrote this report also describes other manifestations of a paranormal nature: "An orange and a pear flew across the entire room where R. was standing. The kitchen table was upset without any movement on the part of R. Milk and food were thrown off the table and stove. The breadboard was thrown on to the floor. Outside the kitchen a coat on its hanger flew across the room; a comb flew violently through the air and extinguished blessed candles; a Bible was thrown directly at the feet of R., but did not injure him in any way" (p. 2, J.R.).

Before I proceed with the dated sequence of events that are related by the Jesuit who reported the entire exorcism, it is important to note that the writer of the report wants to make sure that his account will not be taken by readers as a figment of his imagination, but as a record of true events that took place. Therefore, he provides a list of 14 people who can ascertain that the events took place. Among them he includes the Lutheran ministers who participated in the case, medical doctors and a priest who participated in the exorcism. However, in this same section, he admits that one of these witnesses did not believe in the phenomena.

Witnesses of the Phenomena

To strengthen the validity of his documented exorcism, the author of the Jesuit Report, includes a section of witnesses that were present since the beginning of the ordeal. The report describes this witness section: "Since the beginning of the above-enumerated incidents there have been fourteen different witnesses to testify and verify different phenomena. Two Lutheran Ministers were called in on the case. One of the Ministers invited the boy to his home and slept in the same bed with him. During the night the clawing sounds were heard as they were in R's home. The Minister prayed but the action became stronger. R. was tied to a chair, and the chair tipped over. A psychiatrist was consulted but declared that he did not believe in the phenomena" (J.R., p. 3).

Now the author of the Jesuit Report provides the list of witnesses that were present before the display of paranormal like phenomena. As he relates: "Different displays were witnessed by two aunts of the boy, four uncles and four cousins in St. Louis. The printing 'No School,' was seen by four different people. The swaying of the mattress, the upsetting of the bedroom furniture and the scratching on the mattress were observed by the entire group. March 9, 1949, the violent moving of the mattress and the scratching on the boy's body was observed by the mother, an aunt, an uncle, a cousin of college age, a friend of the family, and by Father Raymond Bishop."

The writer of the Jesuit Report includes the names of the priests who witnessed the adolescent being possessed by the Devil.

Jesuits who saw R under possession:

Rev. George Bischofberger, SJ
Raymond J. Bishop, SJ
Joseph Boland, SJ
William S. Bowdern, SJ
Edmund Burke, SJ
John O'Flaherty, SJ
William Van Rob, SJ
Mr. Walter Halloran, SJ
Prof. Albert Schell, SJ

The Detailed Daily Account of the Exorcism in St. Louis

In the next sequence of events, the writer of the Jesuit Document provides a dated day-by-day report of the major events that took place during the exorcism until after the adolescent was freed from demonic possession.

Monday, March 7, 1949

A close relative, Ronald's aunt, had died recently and the family was somehow convinced that the phenomenon was being caused by this deceased aunt. Therefore, in order to find out, on March 7, while at the home of their relatives, the family held a séance in which letters of the alphabet were placed successively on the top of a porcelain table. Then questions were asked of the spirits by the participants, regarding who was causing the phenomena surrounding Ronald. They were able to piece together a message that indicated that it was a deceased aunt who inhabited the boy's body and was causing these phenomena. The Jesuit Report describes the séance event as follows:

> Home of R's non–Catholic aunt and uncle. Five or six relatives present. Spirit questioned through an alphabetical medium, on porcelain kitchen table.
> Letters of alphabet written on paper were underlined whenever the table moved. A code of messages became evident. Phenomena indicated that the spirit was not the devil but the soul of deceased XXXXXXXX. Spirit confirmed to all present that she was XXXXXXXX by moving a heavy bed two or three feet with no one of the bystanders near the bed. The entire group saw this action.
> Furthermore, writing appeared on R's body while he was reading a comic book. There was a sharp pain. The writing was done through his clothes. When retired, there was violent shaking of the bed and scratching on the mattress. Hardly any relief through the night (J.R., p. 4).

Tuesday, March 8, 1949

During Ronald's family's stay in St. Louis, relatives also witnessed some other strange events. Some of them saw the bed shaking while the boy was lying on it, and also heard scratching coming from his mattress. Furthermore, other marks appeared one day on his body while he was reading a comic book. On Tuesday, March 8, the shaking of the mattress continued. A stool, which was several feet away from the bed, was seen overturned by Ronald's cousin, who spent that night with him. The Jesuit Report describes the event as follows: "At the home of R's Catholic aunt, two cousins and non–Catholic uncle. Shaking of mattress, scratching, stool upset several feet away from the bed. Phenomena observed by cousin who spent the night with R. Mattress continued to move in the direction of the uprights of the bed, even when cousins lay along-side of R. All other members of the family observed the violent shaking of the mattress and heard the scratching sound" (J.R., p. 4).

Wednesday, March 9, 1949

In the meantime, another of Ronald's cousins, who was a student of Father Raymond Bishop at St. Louis University, invited the priest to visit her house and take a look at Ronald. He agreed to see him, suggesting that during his visit it would be a good idea to bless the house and particularly the room where Ronald used to sleep. He also brought over a saintly relic, which was pinned on Ronald's bed, as he thought that the blessing of the house and the relic might stop the phenomena he had been told were taking place around the boy. However, the poltergeist-like dramatic phenomena continued in spite of the relic. As described in the Jesuit Report:

> At home as of Tuesday, Father Bishop blessed the entire house and used a special blessing in R's room and on his bed. A second class relic of St. Margaret Mary was

safety-pinned to the extreme corner of R's pillow. Shortly after R. retired the mattress on his bed began to move back and forth in the direction of the bed uprights. The boy lay perfectly still, and did not exert any physical effort. The movement in one direction did not exceed more than three inches; the action was intermittent and completely subsided after a period of approximately fifteen minutes. When Father Bishop sprinkled St. Ignatius Holy Water on the bed in the form of a Cross, the movement ceased quite abruptly, but began again when Father stepped out of the room. During the course of the fifteen minutes of activity a sharp pain seemed to have struck R. on his stomach and he cried out. The mother quickly pulled back the bed covers and lifted the boy's pajama top enough to show zigzag scratches in bold red lines on the boy's abdomen. It should be remarked that during the fifteen minutes the boy was not out of view of six observers. When the mattress shaking subsided, there was peace for the remainder of the night, i.e., after 11:15 p.m. (J.R., p. 4).

Similar to the placement of the relic on Ronald's pillow, William Friedkin, the director of *The Exorcist*, included a scene in which the mother finds a crucifix under Linda Blair's pillow at the initial stage of the possession.

Thursday, March 10, 1949

The mattress shook again, and the scratching beat out a rhythm as of marching soldiers. Moreover, the relic appeared to have been thrown on the floor. According to Ronald's own words, while he was lying on the bed, the safety pin on the relic of St. Margaret opened, and the relic rose from the pillow, sailed across the room, and struck a mirror. However, the mirror did not break. As described in the Jesuit Document: "Same place as Tuesday and Wednesday. Same people present in the home as of Wednesday with the exception of Father Bishop. Shaking of mattress, and scratching which beat a rhythm as of marching soldiers. Second-class relic of St. Margaret Mary was thrown on the floor. The safety pin was opened but no human hand had touched the relic. R. started up in fright when the relic was thrown down" (J.R., p. 5).

Friday, March 11, 1949

The sequence of events indicated that some of the boy's relatives had arranged to bring Father Bowdern to see Ronald. Father Bowdern decided to take with him, for his visit to Ronald's relatives, a first-class relic of St. Francis Xavier, along with a Novena blessing. He also brought other relics as well: "Same here as above. Same observers as of Thursday with addition of Fathers *********** and Bishop. Father Bowdern had concluded the *** service in the ********** at 9:00 p.m. It was arranged that relatives of the boy would take the two above-mentioned Priests to the home of R. Since the ****** ***** **** In honor of St. ******* Xavier, Father Bowden, the Pastor, thought it proper to take the first-class relic of Xavier along for a Novena Blessing. He likewise carried a crucifix containing first-class relics of several of the North American Martyrs and of St. Peter Canisius" (J.R., p. 5).

Sometime after Father Bowdern arrived at the house, Ronald retired to sleep around 11:00 p.m. Father Bowdern then went into Ronald's room, read the Novena prayer of St. Francis Xavier, and blessed Ronald with the relic. He also placed the crucifix under Ronald's pillow. Then the relatives and the priest left Ronald's room. Shortly afterwards, a loud noise came from Ronald's room. The relatives and the priest rushed in. They found a heavy bookcase in the room turned in a complete circle, and a bench turned over. They also saw the crucifix propelling itself across the room and another relic moved to the foot of the bed. Ronald's bed, which was shaking, stopped only when the observers shouted, "Aunt Dorothy, stop!" The aforementioned event constitutes one of the major differences between *The Exorcist* and the real story in Mount Rainier, where the causal explanation was that the deceased aunt was responsible for the poltergeist-like phenomena. In the film, a demon appears as the actual being responsible for the possession and the surrounding phenomena. The Jesuit Report describes the event as follows:

> Fathers Bowdern and Bishop arrived at the home of R at 11:45 p.m. Before the arrival of the Priests that evening the bookcase in R's room was moved away from the wall quickly and with precision. (The bookcase with books would weigh more than fifty pounds.) Then again just before the Fathers went upstairs to R's room, a quick, scraping noise was heard. The bookcase had swung around from the wall to the side of R's bed in an arc of five or six feet. Father Bishop replaced the bookcase, and then Father Bowdern blessed R. with the relic of St. Francis Xavier and Holy Water. The Fathers prayed the Rosary aloud and then prayed silently from 12:00 to 3:00 a.m. R. had a very normal sleep and there were no manifestations of an evil spirit (J.R., p. 6).
>
> After the above blessing the group of observers went downstairs to review some of the history of the case, when a loud crash was heard in R's bedroom. The boy was dozing when the bottle of St. Ignatius Holy water was thrown (J.R., p. 5).

The Hidden Money of Aunt Dorothy

Ronald's mother hypothesized that all the strange phenomena surrounding her son, were caused by her deceased sister-in-law Dorothy. She truly believed that Dorothy was at the bottom of the strange occurrences taking place with her son. She considered that it probably had something to do with money. There was a belief among the family members that she had left some money in a metal box, hidden somewhere in the house before she died. Therefore, the family decided to conduct a séance to reach out to the deceased aunt and find out about the money. During the séance, they asked the deceased aunt where she had hidden it. In response to the questions, the bed would shake and thump. Then someone would shout, "Dorothy, stop!" and the shaking of the bed would stop momentarily, as though the aunt was hearing the exhortation. Through the dialogue, they believed, the aunt would guide them to find a map that, according to some family members, she had hidden in the attic. The map would lead them to the metal box containing the money, which had been destined for one of her daughters. There is no record, however, as to whether or not the family was successful in finding the map and the money. The Jesuit Report relates the event as follows:

> There is some question about an amount of money which was concealed by Aunt xxxxxxxx before she died. Through many different questions it seemed that the map, which would locate the money hidden in the metal strong box, would be found in the attic of xxxxxxx's home, but only xxxxx the father of R who lives in xxxxxxxxxxxxxxx could find it. When xxxxx's name was suggested, the bed shook violently.
>
> Further questioning revealed that the money was for xxxxxxxxxx, the daughter of xxxxxxxxxx. Whenever the ****** wanted the bed shaking to stop they called, "xxxxx, stop," and the bed stopped as though xxxxxxxxx were listening for a question.
>
> On the night that xxxxxxxx died, she told everyone in the house to go to bed at 10:00 p.m. and she died between 2:00 and 2:30 the following morning. The ****** parallel indicated is that the bed shaking and noise always ceases by **** a.m.

7

Jesuits in Action
The Masters of Exorcism

The Initiation of the Exorcism

Wednesday, March 16, 1949

Permission was granted by the Most Reverend Archbishop Joseph E. Ritter that Father William S. Bowdern, S.J., Pastor of the College Church in St. Louis might read the prayers of exorcism according to the Roman Ritual. Father Bowdern, Bishop, and Mr. W. Halloran, S.J., arrived at the xxxxxxxx home between 10:15 and 10:30 p.m. Shortly after 10:30 R. was sent to bed and Father Bowdern helped him examine his conscience and make an act of contrition. Then Father Bishop, Mr. Halloran, R's mother and the uncle and aunt of R were called into the bedroom in order to prepare for the exorcism. All those present knelt down besides R's bed and acts of Faith, Hope, Love and Contrition were recited together (R said the prayers too) (Jesuit Report, p. 7).

Next Father Bowdern in surplice and stole began the prayers of exorcism. R was awake and the overhead light in the bedroom was kept burning. R kept his hands outside the bed covers. On the first "Praecipio" there was immediate action. Three large parallel bars were scratched on the boy's stomach. From then on ** *** **** of Our Lord and His Blessed mother, and St. Michael scratches parallel on the boy's legs, thighs, stomach, back, chest, face and throat. Those scratches were sharply painful, and caused red marks on the body, and the marks raised up above the surface of the skin, similar to a very slight laceration and caused a small amount of blood to flow. This scratch appeared on his left leg. R. recoiled **** evident, pain as *** mark was made. R. ***** *** that some of the marks felt like thorn scratches, others like brands. The brand marks were the more painful (J.R., p. 7).

In the film *The Exorcist*, while Father Karras and Father Merrin performed the exorcism, scratches appeared spontaneously as they sprinkled holy water over the girl's levitating body. This phenomenon, although less dramatic in

49

the film than in actuality, is still one of its most dramatic scenes, since it appears spontaneously and in the moment.

More Dramatic Demonography: Words and Images

> The most distinct markings on the body were the picture of the devil on R's right leg and the word "HELL" imprinted on R's chest in such a way that R. could look down upon his chest and read the letters plainly. The imprint of the devil and "HELL" appeared at the repetition of the "Praecipio" demanding the evil spirit to identify himself. The devil was portrayed in red. His arms were held above his head and seemed to be webbed, giving the hideous appearance of a bat. All the room observers agreed that the above two signs could not be mistaken for other designs. In further answer to the prayer "Praecipio" two letters "GO" and a third pointed away from the crotch, and indication which might have meant that the devil would leave by way of urination or excrement (J.R., p. 7).

Ronald was branded many time during this exorcism that night, on the stomach, chest, temple, throat, thighs, calves, and back. One branding, which ran from the upper thigh to the clavicle, ruptured his skin and drew blood, while the boy reacted violently and a torrent of profanities flowed from his mouth, along with incredible amounts of spittle. Even though the exact profanities voiced by the possessed adolescent are not known in the actual case, in the film these are quite dramatic; at one point, for example, the female adolescent says that the mother of Father Karras "sucks cocks in hell." The film's profanities include a sort of offensive sexual language that was reportedly not present in the profanities voiced by the actual adolescent boy.

> To the question, posed by the exorcist as to how many demons possessing the adolescent? A single line was scratched on R's right leg. There were at least four heavy brand marks in the form of an "X." This impression may have indicated that the exorcism would take ten days, or that the devil would depart at 10:00 o'clock. At least during the first days of the exorcism the "X" had no significance. The markings on the legs seemed to be long scratches with no special meaning. Marks were made on the boy's body more than twenty-five different times during the course of the evening, each mark causing the boy to double up with pain (J.R., p. 8).

The Third Sign of Possession: Superhuman Strength

At other times, Ronald showed signs of superhuman strength. According to Thomas Allen, the author of *Possessed*, there were moments during the exorcism when 10 people were needed to hold him down. The Jesuit Report does not indicate that 10 people were needed to hold him down, although Ronald needed to be pinned down to the bed. As the Jesuit Report relates:

"From 12:00 midnight on, it was necessary to hold R during his fights with the spirit. Two men were necessary to pin him down to the bed. R. shouted threats of violence at them, but vulgar language was not used. R. spit at his opponents many times. He used a strong arm whenever he could free himself, and his blows were beyond the ordinary strength of the boy" (J.R., p. 8).

In the film *The Exorcist*, the manifestation of this sign of possession or superhuman strength is also apparent, when Father Damian Karras tries to hold down Regan MacNeil, so that Father Lankester Merrin can proceed with the exorcism; even though the girl had loosened the straps tying her down, she was still able to push Father Karras away from her.

Another instance of Ronald's apparent superhuman strength took place while he was sitting in the back seat of a car. According to witnesses, Ronald broke the rib of one of his handlers, and then dove to the front seat, grabbed the steering wheel, and attempted to catapult the car into a river. The car then struck the guardrails as it zigzagged across the traffic lanes.

Friday, March 18, 1949

R. had a spell about 1:00 p.m. His father held him tight in his arms while the mother and aunt prayed the Rosary. The struggling ceased in about one-hour. Fathers Bowdern, Bishop and Mr. Halloran, SI, arrived at R's home at 7:00 p.m., chatted and played a game with R. He retired at 8:15 p.m. R prayed the Rosary with the clergy at his bedside. The novena prayers to Our Lady of Fatima were recited in common. Next the Fathers began the Litany of the Saints, as indicated in the exorcism ritual. In the course of the Litany, the mattress began to shake. R. was awake. The shaking ceased when Father Bowdern blessed the bed with Holy Water. The prayers of the exorcism were continued and R. was seized violently so that he began to struggle with his pillow and the bed clothing. The arms, legs, and head of R. had to be held by three men. The contortions revealed physical strength beyond the natural power of R. R. spit at the relics and at the Priests' hands. He writhed under the sprinkling of Holy Water. He fought and screamed in a diabolical, high-pitched voice. During one of his quieter reactions he was moving his feet in rhythmical fashion. Father Bowdern held the Blessed Sacrament three or four inches from the sole of the moving foot. The movement stopped on the foot which was nearer the Blessed Sacrament. This manifestation of the power of the Blessed Sacrament showed up time after time without fail (J.R., pp. 9–10).

Saturday, March 19, 1949

The exorcists arrived at R's home at 7 p.m. R retired at 8 p.m. and the routine of the exorcism was begun again. Violent shouting with fiendish laughter were a part of the phenomena. The shouting resembled the barking of a dog, and the snapping of R's teeth was truly diabolical. It should be stated again that the violent reactions always followed upon the prayers of the exorcism. There had been no violence from the boy before the exorcism was begun on the night of March 16. When the exorcist asked for a sign through the prayer "Praecipio" on three or four different occasions R urinated, seemingly without control. He complained upon awaking that the urine burned him. Previous to the urination R doubled up with pain in his stomach and he woke up crying. He complained too that his throat hurt him. Songs were sung very beautifully in a clear voice and with real finesse. The best rendition was the "la" of the "Blue Danube" with excellent and flowing gestures of interpretation. Another song was the hymn "The Old Rugged Cross." The striking thing about the singing on this night was the professional ability shown. R cannot sing well in normal life, nor does he like to sing.

Father Bishop hummed the tune of the "Blue Danube" after R was awake, but R was unable to carry the melody. He said he did not know the song. He made this same affirmation several days later (J.R., p. 11).

In the movie *The Exorcist*, the spiting phenomena take place when Father Lankester Merrin begins the exorcism and Regan's first reaction is a spitting or some sort of vomiting that lands on the lens of the exorcist's glasses. Also, the manifestation of Regan's uncontrolled urination takes place at a party, at her mother's house, where she appears in front of the visitors and urinates standing in front of them.

The Exorcism at the Alexian Brothers Hospital

Monday, March 21, 1949

Father Bowdern began negotiation to take Ronald to the Alexian Brothers Hospital since Ronald's family was feeling mentally and physically drained with the procedure. As the Jesuit Report relates: "R was losing sleep, and the mother had to be taken to a physician, so it was thought best to take R to a hospital so that the other members of the family might relax. Since R was so boisterous in his tantrums, it was decided that the Alexian Brothers would have a room away from the regular patients where R could scream without harm to the rest of the hospital" (J.R., p. 12).

Wednesday, March 23, 1949.

During the performance of the ritual of exorcism by the priests, Ronald in a violent reaction broke the nose of father Walter Halloran, member of the exorcist team. Also, he declared that he saw one of the priests in hell. As the Jesuit Report relates:

[I]mmediately upon the first invocations of the Litany R went into his tantrum. He fought and kicked, and spit so that three men could scarcely hold him. In the course of the evening R broke Mr. Halloran's nose and caused Father Roo's nose to bleed. The first blows were accurate, quick, and deadly, although R's eyes were shut. At the "Praecipio" R urinated rather copiously and on coming to himself complained of the burning sensation. There were four or five such urinations during the evening. Sev-

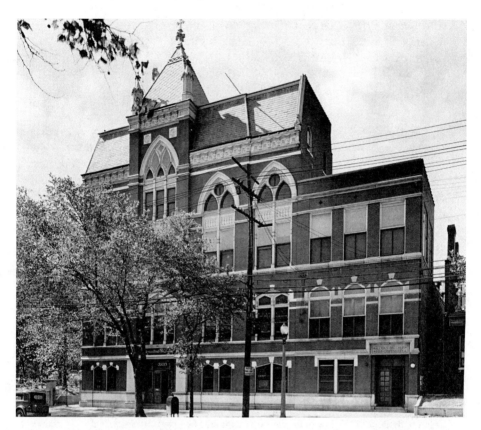

The exorcism ended at the Alexian Brothers Hospital in South St. Louis. The room where it took place was sealed off for years, and that wing of the hospital was demolished in 1978 (SLU Photo Collection-Archives, St. Louis University Libraries, St. Louis University, St. Louis, Missouri).

eral times there was passing of wind through the rectum. The language of R became abusive and dirty. He met one of the Fathers in hell and stated the year as 1957. He indicated surprise at finding the Father in hell. The vile and filthy talk which followed makes anyone shudder. R spoke of his so round, [word, marked out] so firm with a red [words marked out]. He pulled the towel from his loins and shook his body in a suggestive and shimmy fashion. His expressions were lowly and smacked of the abuse of sex. When R came to normal from time to time he would say that the men down there were using filthy language. R was never accustomed to filthy expressions in his regular life. With more contortions, barking and singing R finally went off into natural sleep at 2:30 a.m. His body was limp and completely fagged out (J.R., p. 13).

In the movie *The Exorcist*, a similar event takes place with father Damien Karras, who initiated the investigation of the signs of demonic possession with Regan Teresa MacNeil. During one of the sessions the possessed adolescent tells father Damien Karras that his mother is "with us": "Your mother sucks cocks in Hell, Karras, you faithless slime."

Thursday, March 24, 1949

In this day of the exorcism, some signs appear to indicate to the exorcists that the devil is about to leave Ronald's body. The filthiest talk so far in the ordeal is used by the ostensibly possessed Ronald. As the Jesuit Report relates: "The exorcism was still being conducted at the rectory of the church and Father Wiliam Bordern suspected that one of the marks, the 'X' that appeared on Ronald's body meant that the Devil would leave his body in 10 days."

At the rectory, reactions began at 9:45 p.m., and continued until 2:30 a.m. Father Bishop thought that this would be the last night since it was the feast of St. Gabriel, and the next day was the feast of the Annunciation. Father Bowdern believed that the "X" mark on R from the first night of the exorcism should be interpreted as the 10th day, so he did not expect the devil to leave until the following night.

> R had great physical strength. Four men were holding him. R ran the gamut of shouting, screaming, barking, singing, kindly expressions, urinating, and passing foul air. One of the assisting Fathers was met in hell in 1956. He was called a big fat ass and an ox. Michael, the workman who helped R was constantly in R's bitter imprecations, or in silly rhymes, "Michael, pickle, like sickle.... Michael, you look so dirty." The filthiest talk was given out after midnight on the Feast of the Annunciation. R spoke often he would say, I turned upon the priests at his bedside, "You have big down [words marked out]. You have [words marked out]." Then followed a sucking sound. He called to the exorcist to "cut out the damned Latin. Get away from me."
>
> About 2:00 a.m., R noted from his tantrum that the bystanders were going to stay to the end. In a coy tone he remarked, "You like to stay with me. Well, I like it too."
>
> The blessed sacrament had no noticeable effect in the course of the night (J.R., p. 14).

Friday, March 25, 1949

> After midnight there was some pitching about, but not for long intervals. Cursed his father and spit at him, and then he kicked at the priests at his bedside. He pushed the nearby chair with his foot several times and finally fell into a deep sleep at 1:00 a.m. This was Friday night, the 10th night since the exorcism was begun. Perhaps the "X" given on the first night was to mean 10 days. On Monday night the XXXXXXXX home was blessed by Father Bowdern. No disturbances occurred Monday, Tuesday, or Wednesday nights, and R was getting back to normal life (J.R., p. 14).

Thursday, March 31, 1949

At 11:30 p.m. R went downstairs and complained that he was feeling ill, and that his feet felt cold, then hot. When the family went up to the bedroom with him the disturbances began. First the shaking of the bed. He began to write on the sheet with his finger, explaining between spells that he seemed to be reading from a blackboard. They were unable to make out what he was writing on the sheet. Then he began to talk, telling what he saw on the blackboard. Notes taken by his cousin are as follows:

I will stay 10 days, but will return in 4 days
If XXXXXXXX stays (gone to lunch)
If you stay and become a Catholic, it will stay away. XXXXXXXX
God will take it away 4 days after it has gone 10 days. God is getting powerful.
The last day when it quits it will leave a sign on my front.
Fr. Bishop—all people that mangle [*sic*] with me will die a terrible death.

Family called Rectory about midnight. Fathers Bowdern and Van Roo arrived at the house at about 1:00 a.m. and Father Bowdern began the rite of exorcism.

At the "Praecipio" R (in a spell) called for a pencil. At this point and frequently at the beginning of subsequent spells he addressed one or both of the two persons: "Pete" (most frequently) and "foe." Taking the pencil, he began to write with it on the head of the bed, which was covered with a white cloth.

This type of spell and writing was repeated perhaps eight or ten times. What he wrote was recorded for the most part. The family washed away the writing a few times, making room for more, and XXXXXXXX fastened large sheets of wrapping paper to the bed. The following is a record of most of the writings, though it is not complete. Some of the things written were repeated:

1. In answer to the first set of questions he wrote the Roman Numeral X. (It was clearly the numeral, with crossbars at the top and bottom). This was written four times on this first occasion and was repeated several times during the exorcism, usually in answer to the question, "diem."

2. I will stay 10 days and then return after the 4 days are up.

3. I am the devil himself. You will have to pray for a month in the Catholic Church.

4. (In answer to the command to give "nomen lingua Latina.") speak the language of the persons. (word language was misspelled). I will put in XXXXXXXX's mind when he makes up his mind that the Priests [*sic*] are wrong about writing English.
    I will, that is the devil will try to get his mother and dad to hate the Catholic Church. I will answer in the name of Spite.

5. In 10 days I will give a sign on his chest he will have to have it covered to show my power.

6. He drew a strange thing that looked somewhat like a map, with "2,000 ft." written on it (apparently connected with early dreams about hidden treasure and a map to find it). I believe that it was in this connection that he spoke also, saying "Yeah, this is what I got on the Ouija board." He drew a face also, and wrote the words: "Dead bishop."

7. You may not believe me. Then R will suffer forever.

8. When commanded to give a sign in Latin, he wrote meaningless marks on the paper, not even letters of the Roman alphabet (J.R., pp. 14–16).

Friday, April 1, 1949

The family decided that the baptism of Ronald as a Catholic would help him be free from the devil's possession. As the Jesuit Report reveals:

R had been taking instructions on Catholic doctrine since Wednesday, Mar. 23 under the direction of Father McMahon. R's father and mother leaving R's choice of religion to himself. They had agreed that R would not be confirmed in the Lutheran Church as had been planned previously.

With the relapse into five days of respite the mother, father and R agreed that the proper thing to do was to have R baptized a Catholic. Sponsors were picked and the baptismal party was to arrive at the College Church between 8:00 and 8:30 p.m. As the party of five relatives drove from R's home, R felt a strange sensation in his feet. There were alternations of hot and cold feelings, and the R went into one of his spells. He began by saying, "So you are going to baptize me! Ha! Ha!—And you think you will drive me out with Holy Communion! Ha! Ha!" R grabbed the steering wheel of the automobile and his uncle was forced to pull up to the curb in order to subdue the violence. R stiffened and fought. It was a major task to remove him from the front seat and force him into the back of the car. R's father and uncle held R in the back seat while the aunt drove. Even with careful supervision R leaped up to seize his aunt as she drove. An interesting sidelight is that the radio in the car would not operate while R was in a spell, although it worked before and after.

In the College Church Rectory another hard struggle almost made it impossible for three men to carry R from the car to the Rectory. Inside the door of the Rectory R shouted and spit. He was thrown on the floor of one of the parlors 277 **** [words marked out] his physical violence. Even ice cold water had little effect upon him. The father and uncle were completely exhausted from the battle.

R was carried to the third floor of the Rectory and placed on the bed. There was little hope that the Baptism could be administered at the baptismal font in the presence of the chosen sponsors. Michael, the workman, was chosen as proxy. R was in and out of his seizures for short periods but there was not enough time for the long profession of Faith and abjuration of heresy. Father Bowdern had R repeat the words of a briefer form. Then the regular procedure for the Baptism of infants followed. However, when R was asked, "Dost thou renounce Satan?" he went off into a spell. The action was repeated three or four times, but R went off before he could answer the question with the words, "I do renounce him."

Finally, R was normal long enough to give the answers. When Father Bowdern came to the Baptism proper the physical resistance exceeded any violence of the evening. R remained conscious for the words, "Ego to baptizo in nomine Patris" and then there was a violent upheaval. None-the-less, the Baptism was completed with a generous amount of baptismal water. It seemed from the reactions that the Lutheran Baptism had not been administered properly, or that it had not taken effect.

After the Baptism the prayers of the exorcism were continued. The usual spitting, gyrating, cursing and physical violence continued until 11:30 p.m. (J.R., pp. 16–17).

Saturday, April 2, 1949

R awakened at 9:30 a.m., but was not calm. He threw a pillow at the light and broke the shade and the bulb. The crockery basin in his room was likewise shattered. This was the morning when R was to receive his first Holy Communion. Fathers Bishop and O'Flaherty were called in to assist Father Bowdern in the preparation for Holy Communion. It was evident that the struggle was at hand. There was no difficulty in going through the conditional confession. Perhaps this quietness indicated again that the Baptism of the preceding night had taken effect.

When Father Bowdern began the prayers for the Holy Communion, R went into his spell, kept his eyes shut and his mouth closed, but he was not hard to hold at this time. R rallied for brief moments, yet whenever Father Bowdern brought the Eucharistic particle near R, the boy went into his spell. On five different occasions when the particle was placed in R's mouth, he spit it out onto the corporal or purification, which was always held in front of his mouth for caution.

After nearly two hours of vain attempts Father O'Flaherty suggested that we pray the Rosary in honor of Our Lady of Fatima, especially since this was the first Saturday of the month. When the Fathers had completed the Rosary, another attempt was made with the Holy Communion. This time R was able to swallow and he made his first Holy Communion under extraordinary opposition.

R finished dressing himself and prepared to leave for home. Father Bowdern asked Father O'Flaherty to drive the car while he himself, R's father and R sat in the back seat. It was about 11:45 a.m. Only a few minutes after the car was in motion R jumped up off the seat and grabbed Father O'Flaherty and had to be pulled off with force. R was not normal on the road for more than a few minutes at a time.

At home he came to long enough to eat a fairly good-sized breakfast. During the remainder of the day there were only brief intervals of consciousness. The Sacraments had stirred up Satan more than any other priestly administration. The family was nervously worn from the long day of fighting. Fathers Bowdern, Bishop, O'Flaherty, and Michael arrived at R's home at 7:40 p.m. Spells continued. There was no response to the "Praecipio" before 8:40 p.m. One short spell of less than a minute occurred between 8:40 and 11:15 p.m. During this period R ate a dish of ice cream.

At 11:15 R ran downstairs and sat on the arm of a parlor chair. He was becoming so nervous that he could scarcely stay in the bedroom. Father Bowdern feared that R would become violent downstairs so he asked R to go back to the bedroom. R trotted up the stairs in a boyish fashion, turned into his bedroom and ran straight for the reliquary of the Holy Cross. Father O'Flaherty caught his hand in time, but R reached for the open ritual and tore four pages out of the Exorcism formula. He grasped with lightning speed.

Then followed a spell in which Father Bowdern commanded that R should respond in Latin to the "Praecipio,"—"Dicas mihi nomen tuum, et horam exitus tui finalis." The only responses were a repetition of the Latin words followed by a remark, "or by "No!," or by a laugh of ridicule.

At 12:15 spells continued with the same type of responses to the "Praecipio." There was jumbled mockery of the Latin questions. However, at this stage writing appeared on the boy. The letters "GO" were printed in red as they were on the first night of the exorcism. At the command, "dicas mihi tiem," three parallel scratches appeared on R's thigh. At "horam" an X was branded. Three **8* were branded on different parts of R's body.

At 1:15 a.m., R was so nervous that he begged to get out of bed and sit on a chair. His hands trembled in a nervous frenzy. He begged his father to take him back to Washington on Sunday; he could not stand the ordeal any longer; he feared going crazy. Relief came at 1:40 in a natural sleep (J.R., pp. 17–18).

Sunday, April 3, 1949

At 7:00 a.m., R threw a pillow against the ceiling light, but then went back to sleep. There was another short seizure at 8:30, but R went back to sleep until 11:30, then took breakfast.

About 12:00 noon, R walked downstairs but went into spells several times, but there was nothing of a serious note until 4:00 p.m. R engaged in a ball game with his father, two uncles, and a cousin. At one point he tried to throw the ball to his father, but began to stagger as a drunken man. His father rushed to his assistance when the boy began to run in a straight line across the lawns of two of the neighbors. He ran with his eyes shut and with high speed. Three men closed in on him and carried him back home. In the kitchen R lifted the heavy kitchen table with one of his legs.

R ate very little supper and seemed abnormal. On one occasion he wrapped his ??? around a leg of the table and was pulled away by means of strong ???? force. Fathers Bowdern, Van Roo, Bishop and O'Flaherty arrived at the home at 7:00 p.m. Within a few minutes R had a spell in which he grabbed at his aunt and would have torn her dress if several men had not come to her assistance.

R was carried upstairs fighting but came to himself shortly after he was thrown onto the bed. This was Passion Sunday, so the Fathers thought that God would put an end to R's suffering on this night. The exorcism was begun in full but there was no response at the "Praecipio."

One new feature of this evening was a kind of devilish prophecy concerning R's little cousin XXXXXXXX. Shouting and singing in rhythm, R repeated over and over for about ten minutes, "You will die tonight. You will die tonight." It was hard to quiet R by any means but a pillow in his face.

From 9:30 to 12:00 there was no disturbance except snoring and restless sleep. The Fathers departed at midnight, but more trouble began at 12:30. It became necessary to bind the arms of R with tape and to place gloves on his hands. Then he complained of the pain from the adhesive tape and the heat of the gloves. However, when the tape and gloves were removed, R went about his violence again. It was 3:30 before quiet came.

Monday, April 4, 1949

Arrangements were made that the family was to go back to Washington, D.C., by train at 9:30 a.m. R's father had lost a lot of time from his work, and the strain upon the St. Louis XXXXXXXX [family] was beginning to take its toll. Fathers Bowdern and Van Roo were to accompany R and his parents on the trip.

It was difficult to rouse R from his sleep, but cold water dashed in his face brought him out sufficiently so that he could be dressed. He was taken to the railroad station accompanied by his father, mother, uncle and friend of the family. There was no difficulty boarding the train. R walked and chatted normally. What happened on the trip and thereafter will form another report.

8

Case Study of an Exorcism

Part II

Continuation of Case Study Including the Trip to Washington, D.C., and the Return to St. Louis

Monday, April 4, 1949

En route to Washington there was no trouble on the train all day. One short spell of violence occurred when R retired at 11:30 p.m.

Wednesday, April 5, 1949

R awoke normally on the train and was taken to his home in Maryland without a mishap. In the course of the morning Fr. Bowdern met Fr. Hughes, the assistant pastor at St. James Church at Mt. Rainier, and found that he had made arrangements with the Chancellor of the Archdiocese of Washington that Father Bowdern would have full permission to continue with the exorcism. Neither the Pastor nor the assistant at St. James, in whose parish R lives, was able to assume the full responsibility of the case because of lack of room for the boy. It was thought advisable by all concerned that R should not be kept at home. Fathers Bowdern and Hughes tried several hospitals in Washington, but because of the nature of the case no one was willing to accept the burden.

Wednesday, April 6, 1949

Fathers Bowdern and Hughes drove to Baltimore to inquire about a room at the 77*** Institute. The Daughters of Charity were willing to take the boy but the Doctors objected since the case was not psychiatric, and furthermore, since the hospital was dependent upon the State of Maryland for aid, each*** client had to be accounted for on the records. It would have been strikingly *** to include the treatment of exorcism.

With disappointment in Washington and Baltimore, Father Bowdern decided to call again on his devoted friends, the Alexian Brothers in St. Louis. He called long

59

distance and was assured a place for R through the kindness of Brother Rector (Cornelius).

R was normal during the entire day. He took some exercise in the afternoon. Upon retiring he had one very slight spell which lasted only seconds and may have been a nightmare.

Thursday, April 7, 1949

At XXXXXXXX, R was normal all day. He worked in the afternoon, spaded a little and cut the lawn. But the evening spell lasted for five hours, from 9:15 p.m. to 2:15 a.m.

Branding: R was awake. During the exorcism at the "Praecipio" at least twenty brands appeared on R's body. Many occurred at the name of Jesus as he recited the Hail Mary. The first mark was clearly a number "4." Some other marks may have been the number "4" also, but were obscure. Other marks: single stroke, double stroke, seemingly a pitch fork, several times four strokes or claw marks of various lengths on belly or legs. One set of such claw marks from thigh to ankle tearing off a scab near the ankle. When these marks occurred, the boy's hands were kept away from his body. One branding occurred on his leg just as he started to lie down after the preceding mark had been observed. Most of the branding occurred under his clothing or at least under the sheet covering him.

> Spitting, violence.
> Singing: humming the "Ave Maria."
> Filthy talk.
> Writing on his own body with fingernail the words "Hell" and "Christ" in large capital letters.

Through R the devil said he would keep the Priests until 6 a.m. He made this statement at 2 a.m. when everyone was fagged out. He said he would prove his threat by having 4 awaken immediately. R awoke with a start, but the Fathers were [unintelligible] when sound sleep came fifteen minutes after 2 a.m. It [??] throughout the possession that whenever R was completely [??] God permitted him to go off to sleep and … [???]

Friday, April [8], 1949

R was normal all day. There was a five-hour session in the night from 8:15 p.m. to [??] a.m.

1. Began when R was alone in the bathroom, a few minutes after the Priests (**). Two and one-quarter hours of great physical violence. Half hour of crying. This continued with shorter spells until 1:20 a.m.: violence, spitting, nonsense jumbling of Latin questions, singing Blue Danube, Ave Maria, and so forth. There was filthy talk and movements and filthy attacks on those at the bedside concerning masturbation and contraceptives, sexual relations of Priests and Nuns.

2. Irritated and impatient after the long struggle. Fathers Hughes and Canning arrived with the Blessed Sacrament about 11 p.m. The house was blessed by

Father Hughes. R twice threw pillow in direction of the Blessed Sacrament. He took one sedative, spat it out, then finally swallowed it.

Saturday, April 9, 1949

On the return trip to St. Louis R was normal all day. He underwent a short spell upon retiring in the evening.

Sunday, April 10, 1949

When R returned to St. Louis he was sent immediately to the Alexian Brothers [??] where the Brothers took him into one of their private living rooms for the day. Fathers Bowdern, O'Flaherty, Van Roo, and Bishop arrived at the Hospital shortly after 7 p.m. [???] ... fifth floor where he occupied the same room which was [??] ... visit. The exorcism was completed and several Rosaries [??] but no disturbances occurred.

R went into a good sleep about 11 p.m., but the Fathers decided to awaken him after midnight in order to give him Holy Communion. R was so fatigued that it seemed almost hopeless to keep him awake for more than seconds at a time. When the Fathers were planning to abandon the experiment; R became quite normal and was able to receive Communion without special effort. The Blessed Sacrament brought peace to R. He settled back on his pillow with a smile and was soon in deep sleep. Nothing disturbing happened throughout the night.

Monday, April 11, 1949

Brother Emmet kept R occupied with manual work on his hospital floor, and what was most valuable, won the friendship and confidence of R so that the psychiatric surroundings were more understandable and agreeable.

Fathers Bowdern, Van Roo, Bishop and Mr. Halloran arrived at the Hospital at 8:00 p.m. Father Bishop brought some Catholic readers and stories for R so that he would have more than his catechism for study and reading. R went to bed at 9:00 p.m., and the exorcism was completed. The evening gave every reason for expecting quiet. While the Fathers were reciting the Rosary R felt a sting on his chest, but upon examination only a blotch of red was observable. The Rosary was continued until R was struck more sharply by a branding on his chest. The letters were in caps and read in the direction of R's crotch. "EXIT" seemed quite clear. On another branding, a large arrow followed up the word "EXIT and pointed to R's penis. The word "EXIT" appeared at three different times in different parts of R's body. R felt terrible pains in his kidneys and in his penis. He cried from the burning sensations. When he urinated, he complained of even more severe pain.

At midnight, the Fathers planned to give R Holy Communion, but Satan would have no part of it. Even while the institution of the Blessed Sacrament was explained to R his body was badly scratched and branded. The word "HELL" was printed on his chest and thigh. Upon the explanation of the Apostles becoming Priests and receiving Our Lord at the Last Supper, scratches appeared from R's hips to his ankles in heavy lines, seemingly as a protest to Holy Communion.

When Father Bowdern attempted to give R a small particle of the Sacred Host, the boy was taken off by a quick seizure and the devil said that he would not allow R to receive. After four or five attempts, it was thought that a spiritual Communion would have to suffice. But even the expression of the words "I want to receive You in Holy Communion" was cut off by a seizure at the word "Communion."

From all further indications during the evening, it seemed that the attempts to administer the Sacrament of the Eucharist roused the devil more than ordinarily. He went through his usual routine of fighting, barking, cursing, swearing, spitting and *****, but kept on longer than usual. There was no quiet sleep **** of the edifying events of the night was the devotedness of ****"*** to constant prayer and their professional attitude at the ****.

Tuesday, April 12, 1949

Action began after the exorcism prayers were **** During the general recitation of the Rosary by the ******* Brothers the regular performance began, but with the omission of writing on R's body. The noise and stinging were disturbing to everyone. R gave no response to the "Praecipio" except to imitate the Latin words, then laugh, or say, "Stick it up your ass."

One new phase was the display of the devil's power over the senses and external personality of R. In one instance the devil said he would have R awaken and the boy would be pleasant and attractive. The devil's promise was true. A few minutes later the devil said he would have R awaken, but this time he would be offensive. True to the promise R came out of the spell very irritable and he complained quite bitterly to those who held him.

Several attempts were made to give R Holy Communion after midnight, but each trial was unsuccessful. The devil showed definitely that he was not R speaking, for he said, "I will not let R receive Holy Communion...." It was about 1:30 a.m. before quiet sleep followed.

Wednesday April 13, 1949

R received Holy Communion on arising in the morning without encountering difficulty. During the afternoon R was taken out to the White House (Retreat House) and shown the chapel there, as well as the *"** stations of the Cross. At the fourteenth Station, when R was farthest away from the *********, he went into a spell and had to be carried back to the car by ************. The seizure lasted about twenty minutes.

In the evening R was ready for bed at 8:45. He was bright and cheerful and**************** trick gadgets that Father McMahon had given him. As he sat on the bed, and before any prayers were begun, R went off into a quick but violent seizure. It seemed to the exorcists that this would be an important evening. R spoke almost immediately and said that God had commanded him to leave at 11:00 o'clock tonight, but that he would not leave without a struggle. He proved the latter part of his promise by showing relatively more physical power than at any previous time. He stayed in his first spell for twenty minutes while Father Bowdern worked on the exorcism and the Brothers prayed the Rosary in honor of Our Lady of Fatima. In the

"Praecipio" Father Bowdern had always been ***** in getting response in Latin, and he kept up his demands. The devil ignored the command, answered in pig Latin, playfully imitated the commands, or used the common expression "Stick it up your ass." He began singing the words, "stick it up, stick it up." In no instance up to this point in the case has the devil answered in Latin, although his imitation of Latin was clear and distinct.

Filthy talk and damning threats to those at the bedside continued as on other evenings. A new note of the evening was the loud nuisance shouting of "Fire." At 10:45 R began to imitate the sound of a large church bell sounding out the 11:00 o'clock *****. He sustained the "ng" sound at the end of the word "bong." After 11:00 p.m. the same cathedral bell sounds were repeated, but it was very evident that the devil had deceived everyone by his first remark of the evening.

After midnight unsuccessful attempts were made to give R Holy Communion. Satan said again that he would not permit Holy Communion. He laughed at each of the attempts. R could not repeat the word "Communion," before he went into the spell.

The Brothers had prayed valiantly for several hours around midnight. They completed more than fifty decades of the Rosary and their prayerful assistance is worthy of the highest comment. Round-the-clock adoration of the Blessed Sacrament was begun by the Brothers on Monday or Tuesday evening.

Holy Thursday—Good Friday—Holy Saturday, April 14, 15, 16, 1949.

R received Holy Communion from the Hospital Chaplain, Father Widman, on Thursday morning. The Fathers arrived for prayers of exorcism in the evening. Rosary was continued by the Brothers. There were no reactions before or after midnight on Thursday. The Fathers were informed this night that Brother Rector purchased a new Statue of Our Lady of Fatima and had it placed in a conspicuous spot on the first floor corridor of the Hospital. It was dedicated to the Blessed Virgin with the petition that Our Lady of Fatima would intercede for R in his ordeal. The Brothers promised Community devotions to Our Lady of Fatima should R be spared from further affliction.

No disturbances of any sort occurred on Holy Thursday, Good Friday, or Holy Saturday. R listened attentively to the Tre Ore services broadcast over WEW on Good Friday.

On Holy Saturday, Brother Rector bought a small colorful statue of St. Michael the Archangel. The statue was placed in R's room. It should be remarked here that one of the most effective prayers of exorcism was that dedicated to St. Michael.

After midnight on Saturday, arrangements were made that R should be awakened for 6:30 Communion, and that he should attend the second Mass in the Brothers' chapel, Easter morning.

Easter Sunday, April 17, 1949.

Father Widman, Hospital Chaplain, made three unsuccessful attempts to give R Holy Communion in his room. After some waiting and slapping of R, the fourth attempt succeeded.

Brother Theophane, who was on nurse duty in R's room, was reading the Office of the Blessed Virgin. It was about 6:45 a.m., when he came to the "Regina Caeli" R jumped out of bed, then grabbed the Office Book from the Brother and reached for the scapular from the Brother's habit, which was placed on a nearby chair. R fought and spit at the Brother and trampled the scapular underfoot in an Indian war dance. The devil said, "I will not let him go to Mass. Everyone thinks it will be good for him." It was impossible to get R to the chapel because of his frequent seizures. Father Bowdern was called to the Hospital, and shortly after his arrival the spell was broken. There was no further reaction until evening.

In the evening R was spending a little time with the Brothers at ***** *** outside the Hospital. Brother Emmet was escorting R back to the basement floor of the Hospital when R went into a fighting spell. The Brother was alone and shouted for help but it was some time before the other Brothers heard *** Brother.

Emmet was quite exhausted from the struggle. R was carried into the elevator and placed in his fifth floor room. The Fathers immediately began the prayers of exorcism, and the usual indications of violence continued. The ******showed his power again by saying that he would have R awaken and ask for a knife. He had threatened to kill those who molested him while in his seizure. When R came out of the spell, he asked for a knife so that he might cut an Easter egg.

A little later the devil said that they would have R awaken and ask for a drink of water, and R carried out the plan.

There was no response to the "Praecipio" except taunting remarks to the exorcists. Everyone, including R, was becoming weary of the long performance. R did not begin to sleep until midnight. The Fathers left the Hospital at 12:45 p.m.

9

The Angel of Deliverance
I Command You, Satan, to Leave This Body

Monday, April 18, 1949

8:00 a.m.—R awoke in a spell, kicking at the Brother at the bedside. He jumped out of bed, seized the Holy Water bottle, threatened to throw it at the Brothers, then sprinkled Water toward them. Finally, he threw the bottle over their heads, smashing it against the ceiling.

8:15 a.m.—Father Widman attempted to give R communion, it was impossible. Spitting: unable to make even spiritual Communion: Made one Spiritual Communion. The devil then seized him and said that one devil was out, and that R had to make nine Communions (sacramental or spiritual apparently) and then he would leave his body. R continued for an hour unable to make spiritual communion or to receive the Sacrament.

10:00 a.m.—There were more spells when attempting Spiritual Communion. R was able to say: "I wish to receive you" (That is all the Priest attempted to have him say, since it was sufficient.) The devil laughed and said: "That isn't enough. He has to say one more word, one little word, I mean one BIG word. He'll never say it. He has to make nine Communions. He'll never say that word. I am always in him. I may not have much power always, but I am in him. He will never say that word." Several spells: violence, singing, urination.

11:30 a.m.—R said he was very hungry, and wanted a bath and food. We put him off until noon. Then gave him a tray: cake, ice cream, milk. He threw the glass against the wall, scattering broken glass all over. Violence intermittent until about 1:30 p.m. R was very discouraged and disgusted and mean.

In the afternoon the Brothers brought R a serving of chipped beef and arranged R's tray on a little table in his room. R picked up the plate, ran over to the window, held the plate in an almost perpendicular manner in the palm of his hand and dared the Brothers to step closer. One of the Brothers crawled under the bed to catch R at his feet, the other circled the bed to restrain R's arms, but the plate was fired mightily against the opposite wall. No one was hurt but the plate was broken to bits.

On the trip to the Hospital on this evening the Fathers had decided that in the "Praecipio" Father Bowdern would ask for the responses in English. Moreover, the medals were to be left on R in spite of this protests to the contrary. *** *" * was to be placed in R's hand when he was under his spells. These resolutions were discussed and carried out because of the information gathered from the reading concerning several other cases of possession.

Father Bowdern, O'Flaherty and Bishop arrived at the Hospital at 7:00 p.m. Father Van Roo had been with R during the greater part of the day, but was relieved by the Brothers shortly before the evening meal.

R asked to telephone his mother, but on his way to the telephone he went into a spell and had to be carried back to his room, in a fighting mood.

Father Bowdern read the rite of exorcism quietly. When he came to the words *** *** *****, Tu fiscera regas," he blessed R with signs of the Cross. **" **** *** he repeated the expressions perfectly and asked their meaning. Several times later he repeated the Latin. The signs of the Cross and the Crucifix were very effective. R fought hard when the Crucifix was forced into his hand. In one instance R threw the Crucifix out of his hand.

Next Father O'Flaherty began teaching R the first half of the Ave Maria in Latin because R had expressed a real interest in Latin. In the space of fifteen minutes R could recite a good portion of the prayer unassisted. After the memory lesson, Father O'Flaherty told R the complete story of Our Lady of Fatima to which R paid strict attention. A little later he asked for a Catholic reader containing eighth grade prose and poetry, and then thumbed through several stories as he sat in bed. Finally, in a boyish way, he took to balancing the book on his knees and on his head.

R went into a spell while he held the book on his knees and immediately the book was thrown into the corner of the room. From 9:30 until 10:00 p.m., R was in and out of seizures. During his quiet moments the most impressive prayer of the evening was R's. His reverence seemed truly remarkable.

R was more co-operative this night than he had ever been before. He felt that they had to pray whenever he was out of his seizure. He asked whether he could make Spiritual Communions on his own, and he wondered whether through his prayers he himself could bring on spells at different times. Whenever he became normal he reverted to prayer. He stated several times that he saw more light each time he went into a spell. The light seemed to be at the end of a dark tunnel.

R complained several times that the medals on his neck were hot and he asked that they be removed, but the medal was not taken off. Father Bowdern forced a small reliquary crucifix into R's hand when he was in a spell. The reaction to the medals and the cross was exceptional. When Father Widman blessed R with his ordination crucifix and asked R to kiss the image, R went into a spell.

During all the above seizures Father Bowdern continued the "Praecipio" and asked them the response be given in English. This procedure was a change from the regular routine. In the commands up to this time, Latin had been****** ****. The devil in one instance, March 31, had written that the Priests were*** **** *** Latin answers, and he stated that he uses the language *** *** ***** possessed. While Father Bowdern used the "Praecipio," Father Bishop **** ****** **** *and over again the exorcism prayer ****** ******.

At 10:45 p.m., the most striking event of the evening occurred. R was in a seizure, but lay calm. In clear, commanding tones, and with dignity, a voice broke into the prayers. The following is an accurate quotation:

"Satan! Satan! I am Saint Michael, and I command you, Satan, and the other evil spirits to leave the body in the name of Dominus, immediately,—Now! NOW! NOW!"

Then there were the most violent contortions of the entire period of exorcism, that is since March 16. Perhaps this was the fight to the finish. Father O'Flaherty and the Brothers were weary and sore physically from the exertion. After seven or eight

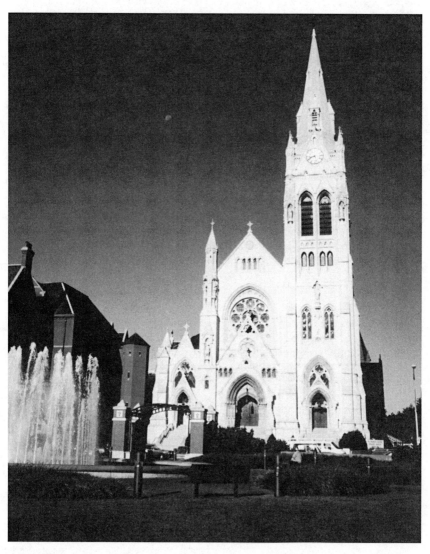

St. Francis Xavier Church on the campus of Saint Louis University. It is said that Saint Michael appeared in the sanctuary when the 1949 exorcism was completed (SLU Photo Collection-Archives, St. Louis University Libraries, St. Louis University, St. Louis, Missouri).

minutes of violence R, in a tone of complete relief, said, "He's gone!" Immediately R came back to normal and said he felt fine.

R now explained what he saw. He said there was a brilliant white light and in that light stood a very beautiful man, with flowing, wavy hair that blew in the breeze. He wore a white robe that fitted close to his body. The material gave the impression of scales. Only the upper half of the body of this man was visible to R, in his right hand he held up a wavy and fiery sword in front of him. With his left hand he pointed down to a pit or cave. R said he saw the devil standing in the cave. R felt the heat from the cave and saw the flames.

First the devil fought, resisting the angel and laughing diabolically. Then the angel smiled at R and spoke, but R heard only the one word "Dominus." As the angel spoke, the devil and about ten of his helpers ran back into the fire of the cave or pit. After the devil disappeared, the letters "Spite" appeared on the bars of the cave. As the devils disappeared into the pit R felt a pulling or tugging in the region of his stomach. As the devils disappeared, he felt a snapping, and then felt relaxed completely. He said that this was the most relaxed feeling he had since the whole experience began in January.

R relates his visual experience at 11:00 p.m. This time was approximate to the time that the manifestations of the devil began in Cottage City, Maryland, on the evening of January 15, 1959.

After 12:00 midnight, R ***led another Rosary and the Fathers and Brothers responded. He was composed and peaceful. Arrangements were made that Father Van Roo, SJ, would say Mass for R in the Hospital Chapel at 9:30, Tuesday morning.

Tuesday, April 19, 1949

The devil is gone!

R was awakened from a heavy sleep and taken to the chapel where he attended the first Holy Mass since he became a Catholic. He likewise received Holy Communion at the altar rail with no difficulty. R promised to say ten Rosaries in thanks giving to Our Lady of Fatima during the course of the day. When the Fathers **** R in his thanksgiving. Since Monday at 11:00 p.m. there have been no indications of the presence of the devil.

Dated the Feast of St. Mark, April 25, 1949.

Followup:

August 19, 1951. R and his father and mother visited the Brothers. R, now 16, is a fine young man. His father and mother also became Catholic, having received their first Holy Communion on Christmas Day, 1950.

11/8/70 Verified residence of XXXXXXXXXXXXXXX with telephone operator xxxxxx lives in xxxxxxxxxxxx xxxxx now lives in xxxxxxxxx Has unlisted phone number.

10

Science in Search
of the Truth
Assessment of the
Mount Rainier Exorcism

In my scientific discussion and analysis of the background of the Mount Rainier Exorcism, information provided by the Jesuit Report as well as the complementary research conducted on the case will be key in the assessment presented in this chapter. The scientific assessment will rely heavily on the model used by John Nicola in his book *Diabolical Possession and Exorcism* (1974)[1] to investigate the causal factors of apparent cases of demonic possession and exorcism. In his approach, Father Nicola, as outlined in Chapter Two of his book, uses a hierarchy of causality model, in which he includes categories briefly described below. I will use these categories to explain the phenomena surrounding the Mount Rainier Exorcism from a scientific standpoint.

1. Fraud and Deception: This category includes those subjective elements that predispose a person to look for preternatural influences as well as tricks and pranks played by others as causal factors related to the phenomena. A person or thing intended to deceive others, typically by unjustifiably claiming or being credited with accomplishments or qualities. For instance, "mediums exposed as tricksters and frauds."

2. Natural Scientific Causes: Under this category, data drawn from physics and psychology are included, depending on whether the phenomena are physical or psychological in nature. For example, noises, rushes of air, coldness, levitation, movement of objects, etc., are physical phenomena for which science might offer an explanation. On the other hand, in this same category we have psychologi-

cal phenomena such as hysteria, hallucinations, seizures, and delusions, which can cause individuals to feel certain that they have
had an extraordinary experience, although there really exists no
objective foundation for it.

3. Parapsychological Causes: In this category, ESP (extrasensory perception) phenomena such as poltergeist occurrences will be considered as a causal factor.

4. Diabolical Influences: This is considered as causality factor since,
for some of the participants in the actual case and for experts on
demonic possession such as John Nicola, we are dealing here with
an "actual" case of demonic possession. According to them, there is
no other explanation to account for the phenomena.

The aforementioned hierarchy of causality factors, which will applied to the
evaluation of the Mount Rainier Exorcism, is based on the "Principle of
Causality"—that is, that every effect must have a proportional cause.

Following Nicola's line of thinking in this regard, given this hierarchy
of possible causes, an investigation must begin with an attempt to rule out
those which are not applicable to the case, looking always for moral certitude
or at least a strong probability. When the elimination of some causes, he
argues, still leaves us with more than one possibility, we act in practice as
though the cause that is highest in the proposed hierarchy is the operative
one. According to Nicola, this is what is considered the "principle of scientific
economy," which states that, when a natural and ordinary explanation is possible, we do not have to resort to unusual and extraordinary causes even
though the potentiality, and the possibility, is always there.

Moreover, continues Nicola, the principle demands that, unless the first
possibilities can be excluded, they are to be considered the causes for practical
purposes. If there should be a preternatural cause involved in this case, it
would be the devil.

The aforementioned principle of science proposed by Nicola is based
on the so-called principle of Occam's Razor, which is often expressed in Latin
as the lex parsimoniae (translating to the law of parsimony, law of economy,
or law of succinctness). William of Ockham (c. 1287–1347),[2] who proposed
the above principle, was an English Franciscan theologian, an influential
medieval philosopher, and a nominalist. His popular fame as a great logician
rests chiefly on the maxim known as Ockham's (or Occam's) Razor. The term
razor refers to distinguishing between two hypotheses either by "shaving
away" unnecessary assumptions or by cutting apart two similar conclusions.
It is defined thus: When competing hypotheses are equal in other respects,
the principle recommends selection of the hypothesis that introduces the
fewest assumptions and postulates the fewest entities while still sufficiently

answering the question. To quote Isaac Newton, "We are to admit no more causes of natural things than such as are both true and sufficient to explain their appearances. Therefore, to the same natural effects we must, so far as possible, assign the same causes." Another interpretation of the razor concept would be that "simpler hypotheses (not conclusions, i.e., explanations) are generally better than the complex ones."[3] In order to make this principle clearer to the reader, we can sum up the principle by saying: The simplest explanation is usually the right one. Detectives use it to deduce who's the likeliest suspect in a murder case—you know, the butler did it. Doctors use it to determine the illness behind a set of symptoms.

For instance, when somebody reports that he or she has been abducted by aliens, instead of explaining that the causality of the abduction is actual aliens, a simpler explanation may be more accurate, such as that this was a dream instead. Obviously, the simpler explanation must be supported by facts. In the Mount Rainier case, the priest ran into a supernatural explanation, the demonic possession hypothesis, by shaving away more likely or simpler explanations such as psychological or psychiatric disturbances that could have been better supported by the facts surrounding the case.

In Nicola's model for investigating cases of demonic possession, the fifth category, or miraculous explanation, is excluded, because he considers that the phenomena involved are of a poltergeist variety and the divine would not be involved in the trivial and foolish. However, it cannot be discarded as a real causal factor if the other four categories do not satisfactorily explain the phenomena surrounding the Mount Rainier Exorcism. At the same time, any supernatural explanation could hardly be proven, so it would remain as a matter of faith in the event that the supernatural hypothesis was to appear to have a strong possibility as an explanatory causal factor.

Thus, following Nicola's line of thinking, this leaves us with only four causal categories within the framework of which the data will be analyzed and interpreted for the Mount Rainier–St. Louis exorcism. The approach that I have borrowed from Nicola is suitable to this particular case, because it permits the inclusion of causal factors in the context of which the demonic agency hypothesis can also be considered as a feasible explanation. Furthermore, some of the features and phenomena of the case could to some extent fit any of the aforementioned hypotheses, thus meeting the criteria of several of the causal factors of Nicola's hierarchy model. For instance, the parapsychological hypothesis was initially considered by the Rev. Luther Schulze, a minister involved in the case, as the most viable hypothesis to explain the phenomena. Similarly, the diabolical agency hypothesis was considered the actual cause of the phenomena by William Bowdern, the main exorcist on the case, and John Nicola himself (Nicola, 1974), who became a consultant to the film *The Exorcist*.

As for the demonic possession hypothesis held by Father Bowdern on the Mount Rainier–St. Louis case, he replied as follows to William Peter Blatty when the author questioned his explanation of the case: "I can assure you of one thing: the case in which I was involved was the real thing [possession]. I had no doubt about it then and I have no doubt about it now" (Bryan, 1982, p. 183).[4]

Obviously, Bowdern's assessment of the case was not based just on a personal belief, since, as an official religious authority, for him to have decided that the Mount Rainier case was a genuine instance of demonic possession, he had to depend on an actual assessment of it based on the evidence required in the Roman Ritual. Therefore, he had to follow the guidelines established by the Catholic Church to diagnose cases of demonic possession. These guidelines are found in the Roman Ritual, which will be discussed later; clearly, for him the case met the requirements established by the Ritual to render a diagnosis of demonic possession. Moreover, he had participated in the actual exorcism and witnessed the phenomena surrounding the case, a situation that strengthened his belief in the demonic possession agency hypothesis.

Others, such as the Catholic theologian Juan Cortes and writer Florence Gatty, who have also evaluated the case in their book titled *The Case Against Possessions and Exorcisms* (1975), hold to the second category hierarchy hypothesis of Nicola's model, which places the causality of the case in psychological mechanisms.

In addition to the aforementioned causality hypotheses relating to the Mount Rainier case, which fit Nicola's model, some more recent findings by Allen (1993) and Rueda (1990–1996)[5] shed new light on the case. Their research and information on the case seem to point toward and fit the first category of the model—that is, the fraud and deception hypothesis—which has not been given serious attention, except by earlier researchers such as John Nicola and Juan Cortes in their evaluations of the case.

As mentioned above, the Mount Rainier–St. Louis case provides us with the whole array of possibilities of the hierarchy of causality postulated by Nicola, in the context of which we can evaluate the new details and data recently uncovered, as previously indicated by the author of this book and writer Thomas Allen in his book *Possessed* (1993). It is important to note that some later findings in the case have presented us with a new hypothesis that was initially not considered very strongly as the main possible cause of the phenomena surrounding it. That is the "fraud hypothesis," which is supported strongly by some of the new findings on the case, although it was not considered or embraced by many involved in it, who with insufficient evidence were very eager to entertain the demonic agency hypothesis. Among them were William Bowdern and some of the other priests involved in the actual exorcism, who rendered a diagnosis of it without much hesitation or research.

In this scientific analysis, the whole array of possibilities from the hierarchy of causality proposed by Nicola will be considered, allowing us to consider and investigate the different possibilities of his model. Fraud, psychological, parapsychological and demonological, will be considered as a plausible explanation for the phenomena surrounding the Mount Rainier case. In this framework or explanatory model, the oldest and newest data on the case can be nicely assessed in order to determine the most likely causality hypothesis of the related phenomena. Therefore, the four hypotheses in the aforementioned hierarchy proposed by Nicola will be discussed below in the context of the Mount Rainier case.

Moreover, following Nicola's rationale that, if we can exclude the first three possibilities of his explanatory model, then the fourth possibility appears as the most likely explanation, we will consider the Demonic Agency Hypothesis as the causal factor. Indeed, if the fourth possibility at the end of this evaluation appears as the most likely hypothesis to explain the case, it will have to be conditioned on the theological premise that the Devil exists, which, of course, cannot be proved, even if the fourth possibility ends up as the most viable explanation. This does not mean that this demonic agency hypothesis can be completely disproved nor denied, but enters into the realm of faith in the Catholic dogma of the existence of the Devil as an independent entity that exists in this world and can possess human beings.

11

The Art of Trickery
The Fraud and Deception Hypothesis

In his book *Experimental Psychical Research* (1963),[1] Thouless states: "The investigator who is rigidly skeptical when he is told stories of the marvelous, must not be foolish and credulous of stories merely because they claim to undermine the marvelous" (p. 25).

When J.B. Rhine, the Director of Duke's University Parapsychology Laboratory, first learned about the Mount Rainier case from the Lutheran minister Luther Miles Schulze (the minister of Ronald's family church whom they consulted for assistance in 1949), he admitted the possibility that such phenomena could have occurred, as reported by the minister. He was not, however, credulous, and took a guarded position. He had not witnessed any of the phenomena and, therefore, considered that perhaps the minister might have had gotten caught off guard when confronted with the unexpected. As indicated by Brian[2]: "He wondered if the Reverend Schulze had unconsciously exaggerated some of the facts, as the most honest and intelligent people may do at times, especially when confronted with the unexpected and the traumatic" (p. 183).

In reply to Schulze's initial account of the phenomena, which he had not witnessed, Rhine declared: "As you know, the most likely normal explanation is that the boy is, himself, led to create the effect of being the victim of mysterious agencies or forces and might be sincerely convinced of it. Such movements of the chair and the bed might, from your very brief account of them, have originated within himself. I presume you observed the movements in good light and were not in any way relying upon his account of it" (April 2, 1949).[3]

Moreover, he warned the Reverend Schulze of the possibility that the phenomena surrounding the boy could have been explained by fraud. He further indicated in a letter addressed to the minister: "Could you give me an account of the first hand evidence you have of these phenomena—what you actually saw the boy do or witnessed in his presence? If I could be entirely sure that the phenomena are not explainable by trickery, conscious or unconscious ... the reason I take this guarded position is that a number of these cases have been reduced to clever trickery, and since we are not ordinarily prepared for the unusual sort (rather, pathological) of faking that is sometimes practiced, we are not as guarded as would be required to see everything that is going on" (April 21, 1949).[4] Dr. J.B. Rhine is therefore the first one to suggest the possibility of fraud and deception in the Mount Rainier case. According to John Nicola (1974), the fraud hypothesis should be the first consideration in searching out the causality of paranormal occurrences, since human beings are very superstitious, which makes us vulnerable to fraud and deception.

In sum, are fraud and deception a plausible explanation in the Mount Rainier Exorcism? With the exception of Cortes and Gatty (1975), little attention has been paid to this possibility by those who have investigated the case, such as Nicola (1974) and, more recently, Allen (1993). Actually, Nicola denies any possibility of fraud in this particular case, as, according to Allen, he believed it was a genuine case of demonic possession.

In denying the possibility of fraud, Nicola in his book *Diabolical Possession and Exorcism* (1974) declares, with regard to some of the phenomena in the case: "They watched the sheets on their son's bed stand out stiffly like a porcupine's quill. Then slowly the mattress with the boy on it levitated off the bed and floated in the air. In the weeks to follow this was to be repeated several times on different beds, both in private homes and in the hospital. I interject this statement as evidence against the fraud hypothesis which might logically come to mind at this time, i.e., that the bed had somehow been rigged with a mechanical device" (p. 109).

J.B. Rhine, concerned that the Reverend Schulze could have been deceived by trickery or fraud as he observed the phenomena, further questioned the priest to make sure that was not so. In a letter[5] dated July 1, 1949, he asked if a light had been on in the room, adding that he "would like to know about where you were located while the chair was overturned."

Although the case sounded to Rhine like a conventional poltergeist attack, he nevertheless suggested to the Reverend Schulze that fraud could be considered a plausible hypothesis to account for the phenomena. Like a good scientist, he wanted Schulze to rule out first any natural explanation, as suggested by the Principle of Scientific Economy or Occam's Razor. As the principle indicates, "When a natural explanation is possible, we do not have to resort to unusual and extraordinary causes"[6]

Rhine's cautious position and reservations regarding the case were entirely justified. It is important to note that throughout history claims of the paranormal have been plagued by fraud. In particular, in those examples in which adolescents have been involved, trickery has often been detected. Among these cases, we have the Columbus Poltergeist, which took place in 1984, in which Tina, the alleged poltergeist agent, was caught at some point playing tricks. For instance, at one point, film shown in slow motion captured what the human eye had missed—that is, Tina quietly moved the objects.

Furthermore, Nicola (1974) declared with regard to mediumship: "My conclusion after a study of spiritualistic mediums was that approximately ninety-eight percent of the alleged phenomena produced by mediums were explained by fraud, deception and perfectly natural events which were imagined to be otherwise. I think that this percentage could be extended to all versions of occultism. Of the remainder, another good portion can be explained by unconscious psychological conditions and by parapsychology. Therefore, only a fraction of one percent really requires a preternatural agency" (p. 36).

It is important to note that the aforementioned assertion about mediums is made by Nicola in the context of a book on demonic possession and exorcism. Does he actually imply that the same percentage holds true also with regard to demonic possession cases? This possibility certainly exists. However, interestingly, he avoids using the term demonic possession in the context of the chapter on fraud and deception. He further concludes: "What I am trying to bring out is that pranksters are numerous.... Realizing how vulnerable we are to deception, we need to be very circumspect about making judgments on the preternatural causality of unusual occurrences" (p. 37). It seems that we can infer from Nicola's chapter on fraud and deception that the term unusual occurrences include demonic possession, even though he avoids stating the connection. Obviously, the indirect assumption made by Nicola in this chapter is that fraud and deception are also a plausible explanation in a rather high number of cases of demonic possession.

So we are left with the question: to what extent were fraud and deception present in the phenomena manifested in the 1949 Mount Rainier/St. Louis exorcism?

The above question needs to be reconsidered in the light of new information that was published by Thomas Allen in 1993 in his book *Possessed*, as well as my own investigation of the case, which includes interviews with some of the participants who were still alive. As previously outlined, included in Nicola's model for the investigation of demonic possession cases was the general category of fraud and deception. Therefore, the fraud hypothesis is first analyzed, highlighting the subjective elements that predispose a person to look for preternatural influences as well as tricks and pranks played by others. Secondly, the more objective elements of the fraud/deception hypothesis will also be evaluated on the case.

Tricks and pranks: Is there any element or phenomenon of the Mount

Rainier/St. Louis case suggestive of fraud? Could some of the phenomena have been manufactured by the possessed—in this case, the boy Ronald? The above hypothesis, this fraud possibility, will be explored in the light of the new information which has arisen as a result of my own extensive investigation of the case for the last 20 years.

Actually, the reason why the Reverend Schulze had invited the 14-year-old boy to his premises and spent a night with him was that he wanted to prove that someone was playing tricks in the case. As Nicola further explained (1974), "He [Reverend Schulze] tried to laugh off the family's 'preposterous story' as a figment of their imagination. On the surmise that someone was playing tricks in the house, the minister decided to keep the boy at the parsonage for a time" (p. 109).

Undoubtedly, Ronald must have had a reason for wanting to play tricks to accomplish his objective of avoiding a noxious stimulus, as part of the story suggests. In this regard, it is important to mention that Ronald had an aunt who lived in St. Louis and often visited the family. This aunt, whom we will call Aunt Dorothy, plays a very important and mysterious role, which may, in turn, explain why Ronald may have manufactured some of the observed phenomena. This mysterious aunt had died shortly after the phenomena surrounding Ronald began to manifest.

Aunt Dorothy was a spiritualist interested in occult practices. Also, she was Ronald's favorite aunt, with whom he had developed a very special and bonding connection. She also treated her favorite nephew as somebody special. Moreover, she had taught Ronald, according to some witnesses on the case, some of her beliefs about communication with the dead, which she believed could be accomplished via the Ouija board.

Evidently, since he was faced with some problems at home with his schooling, it is little wonder why Ronald preferred to live with his aunt in St. Louis. As the Reverend Schulze recalls, "The boy had a favorite aunt and I thought initially that he was doing all these things to attract attention, avoid going to school, get the trip to St, Louis, visit his favorite aunt and obtain other multiple benefits."[7]

The aforementioned hypothesis by the Reverend Schulze is supported by the numerous marks that appeared on the boy's body and that clearly indicated "Go to St. Louis" and "No," when the issue of going to school was brought up by his mother. For instance, a mark appeared on his body while he looked at himself in the bathroom mirror; he screamed, and when his mother rushed into the bathroom, a blood-red message appeared on his skin reading "Go to St. Louis." This indicated precisely the place where he wanted to go to be with his aunt. But why would the entity indicate St. Louis, where the boy's favorite aunt lived, and not New York or some other place in the country? Furthermore, what benefit would the entity obtain from going to St. Louis?

Furthermore, accounts of the event suggest that later marks appeared that indicated not only the place, but also the day for his departure and the length of time that he would have to stay in St. Louis. As Schulze recalls, "The family told me that the word Saturday appeared on the boy's hip, and three and a half weeks in answer to questions regarding the length of time the entity wanted to be in St. Louis."[8] Interestingly, we have here an entity that sets the complete stage for an entire trip, establishing the destination, the time of departure, and the length of stay in St. Louis. A travel agency would not be needed to plan such a complete trip!

Then, when the possibility of sending him to school while in St. Louis was raised with Ronald, a new mark appeared denying such possibility in terms of a blatant "No" mark on both legs. According to the family reports, the skin branding would occur spontaneously on the boy's body in response to questions posed by the mother and when Ronald's hands were visible. His body seemed to be acting as a Ouija board.

The family, according to the Reverend Schulze, was very superstitious and credulous, and decided to obey the messages and body signs produced by an apparently strange force that was tormenting the boy with painful marks and bleeding. The question remained as to why the entity supposedly possessing Ronald would react so negatively towards the possibility of going to school. If the boy was possessed, then we can understand that the entity might be afraid to going to a sacred place such as a church, but why the hostility to school? This seemed more like a human motive rather than a supernatural one.

But the entity is trying by all means to avoid school. In a very definite matter, it manifests itself through the skin marks on the one person who evidently didn't want Ronald to attend school—that is, Ronald! The credulous and superstitious family decided to comply with the messages from the possessing entity.

In sum, it seems plausible that Ronald may have manufactured the marks himself in order to attract attention, visit his favorite aunt, avoid going to school, etc. This hypothesis is supported by the following events: First of all, a close friend of the family indicated that Ronald had expressed interest in going to visit his aunt in St. Louis. Secondly, he had some problems in school with other children, since he was quite introverted. Thirdly, the boy used to play with the Ouija board with some friends at his aunt's house. He often used to say how much he loved his aunt, who had taught him the Ouija board, and that he would gladly go to St. Louis to live with her.

Also, according to "Ida Mae," a close friend of the family, the father played an intriguing role, since Ronald was his only son. He loved him greatly, but there was frequent disagreement regarding his discipline. The mother favored stricter measures to train the boy; however, the father was more inclined to spoil him and sometimes disagreed with the mother's disciplinary actions. Ida Mae indicated that he seldom directly confronted the mother, who had a stronger command of the family's decisions. The mother clearly opposed the idea of Ronald's leaving school and going to St. Louis, probably because he was at the time attending school in the area and a move would mean that Ronald would be interrupting his schooling before the regular semester was over.

Even if she conceded the necessity of the move because of the son's possession, she was still determined that Ronald attend school even in St. Louis. When she proposed such a plan, a blatant "No" mark appeared on the boy's body, rejecting the idea. Why would a demonic entity be so persistent in avoiding a school environment? This surely sounds more like a human desire than a superhuman force possessing the child.

Ida Mae observed, "If there was a decision to be taken regarding important family matters," it was the mother who was in charge. That is, "she had the final word." For instance, as Ida relates, when Ronald wanted permission for something, the father would tell him, "Ask your mother; if she approves, I will approve too." Furthermore, the dynamics of the family relationship revealed, according to Ida, that the mother had a considerable amount of influence over her husband. For instance, if there was an argument or dispute between the two over a family decision, the father would opt not to confront her and would leave her to make the final decision.

The above family dynamics lead to the following tentative conclusions: Ronald strongly desired to move to St. Louis to live with his favorite aunt and thus avoid going to school. His mother opposed the idea on the ground that she did not want him to miss school.

The father may have supported his "spoiled child" in his wish to go to St. Louis, but would not openly take his side in confrontation with the mother, "knowing that she opposed the idea."

Thus, aware that he would not obtain permission from his mother to move to St. Louis via "normal means," even if his father supported him, Ronald decided to play some clever tricks to scare his superstitious mother, since she believed in mediumistic and spiritual séances.

For instance, in his book *Possessed*, Thomas Allen (1993) declared that "Phyllis" would not call herself a spiritualist, but she did believe in some of what "Harriet" professed. Allen refers to the people involved as Robbie (Ronald), Phyllis (Mrs. Hunkeler, the mother of Ronald), and Aunt Harriet (Aunt Dorothy). Aunt Harriet told Robbie and his mother Phyllis that, in the absence of a Ouija board, the spirits could try to get through to this world by rapping on the walls. Therefore, the family was aware of alternative methods for attempting to make contact with the dead. Robbie, who loved his aunt so much, undoubtedly recalled the lessons on spiritualism taught by her and knew the methods by which the spirits communicated with the living.

One example of the mother's susceptibility to being easily convinced by the spirits is when a mark appeared on the boy's body, indicating that they should go to St. Louis. When the mother saw the mark, she immediately decided to follow the advice without further question. As indicated in the Jesuit Report: "One day while Ronald was looking at himself in the bathroom mirror, he screamed, since a mark had appeared across his chest that spelled out 'Louis.' When the mother saw the mark, she immediately told him that they would go to St. Louis right away and set out to make the preparations for such a trip."[9] Since Ronald knew how much his mother believed in spirit communication via rapping, it would not have been difficult for spirits to convince her via even more dramatic means such as marks on her beloved son. Not only were the spirits communicating, but they were also torturing her child. I wonder if any mother would react differently from the way Ronald's mother did, even if she was a natural skeptic.

Another interesting aspect of the case was when a dripping noise was heard at the house when they, Ronald and his mother were by themselves in the grandmother's bedroom. When they entered the room listening to the loud dripping, a painting of Christ hanging on the wall began to shake, as if the wall had been bumped. Furthermore, when Ronald's parents arrived later, there was a very definite scratching sound under the floorboards near the grandmother's bed. From that night on, scratching was heard every night around the same time (seven o'clock) and would persist until midnight.

These events can be explained in the context of fraud. One hypothesis is that Ronald may have received some help from his father in order to reinforce his message to his reluctant mother. Even though this may sound preposterous at first, it has to be considered in terms of Nicola's model, as long as there is any possibility that it is true. For instance, Ronald's father was an experienced handyman, very skilled in electrical work and carpentry; therefore, it is conceivable that he may have assisted his beloved son in conveying the message to the reluctant mother. We also have here a man who is very eager to help his child while at the same time preferring not to confront his wife directly. Therefore, he may have found it comfortable to convey a simple message to his wife via rapping, which she was very likely to believe. Thus, as preposterous as this hypothesis may sound, it is quite possible that Ronald's father may have helped him set up an electrical mechanical device under the floor of the mother's bed, which could produce scratching sounds.

The psychological dynamics of the family support this hypothesis. First of all, the father was sympathetic to his son's wish to go to St. Louis and he wanted to please him in everything, without confronting his wife. It may have been he who conceived the idea of conveying a few spirit messages that would easily convince his credulous wife to allow Ronald to go live in St. Louis. He actually had the knowledge to create a device to convey the messages. A friend of the family, Ida Mae, described him thus: "He was a handyman, a neat person, very clean. Also, he was very active in the church; he used to do all kinds of work for his local church. For instance, if something needed to be fixed, such as work related to carpentry or electricity, he would do the job. He was so skilled that he even designed some nice wood earrings for one of my birthdays. I remember he made something for the church windows to stop a drop."[10]

Undoubtedly, the father had the technical knowledge to create a device that could produce noises similar to scratching. Such a device could have been placed under the wooden ceiling of the second floor in the grandmother's bedroom, from where the sounds initially came. Moreover, that bedroom was the ideal place to set the device, since, if it had been placed in Ronald's bedroom, he would have been the prime suspect of creating such sounds. The grandmother, who was an old lady with deteriorating hearing, could be more easily deceived.

In support of this hypothesis, we can mention the features of the scratching phenomenon. For instance, the rhythmic scratching sounds had a definite pattern in terms of duration, time of occurrence, and rhythm, that make us suspect that they may have been produced by a mechanical device. With regard to the quality of the initial sounds, such as the dripping heard by Ronald and his grandmother, Thomas Allen[11] relates this event as follows: "When they first heard the sounds, they went into each room and stopped and listened, straining to find the location of the sound." Here we have two people trying to detect a sound that, at a distance, sounded like a dripping noise; however, as Allen further relates, "the sounds became more distinct as they got closer to the source of the sound." In other words, if a mechanical device had been set under the wood floor to produce rhythmic sounds such as scratching, it is quite feasible that such sounds would change in quality when they were at a distance as compared to when they were closer to the source. At a distance, they may have sounded like a dripping noise; however, when closer to the source, they may have sounded like scratching noises.

Furthermore, as previously indicated, they "stopped and listened, straining to find the location of the sound." Clearly, the sound was not very distinct to them at a distance. However, standing near the source of the sound produced a stronger sound effect when they stamped on the floor. If a mechanical device was under the floor and they stamped over it, producing pressure on the device, obviously the quality of the sound had to be distinct. Furthermore, in support of this hypothesis, we can also point to other aspects of the quality of the sounds such as time, duration, and rhythm. Thus, according to the story, the scratching sounds continued for ten days, starting about seven o'clock and fading away around midnight.

This pattern of the phenomenon leads us to suspect that a mechanical device may have been placed under the floor. Another interesting aspect is that the sounds started every day at seven o'clock and faded away at midnight for ten days on a regular basis. But why would the spirits start the phenomenon at a regular time and stop every day around the same time as well? Why for ten days specifically, and at the same time of day? Initially, the family suspected that a rodent was responsible for the sounds and that they were connected to Aunt Dorothy's death. But why would a rodent be so regular in producing sounds for the exact same length of time, in such a rhythmic fashion, for so many hours, and for ten days and no more?

Finally, according to the story, by the time Ronald returned from his few days at the Alexian Brothers Hospital, there was a very definite scratching sound under the floorboards in all the rooms. Does that resemble the behavior of a rodent? Or were the clear and definite sounds on a very regular basis produced by a spirit? Also, if a spirit was connected with the production of the very regular pattern of sounds, why would it be interested in producing these particular sounds?

Interestingly, the sounds stopped on the exact day of the death of Ronald's favorite aunt. Evidently, the news of this death devastated Ronald; it probably left him depressed and discouraged in his attempt to convince his mother to allow him to go to St. Louis. Consequently, the sounds stopped, since there was no longer a benefit to producing them, and the game was now over.

However, there was still another powerful motivation to go to St. Louis, namely, avoiding going to school. It is important to note that, before this ordeal began, Ronald was having some problems at school, which could explain why, in spite of the death of his aunt, he still wanted badly to move to St. Louis. According to Ida Mae, Ronald's mother would not openly discuss his school problems further, even with one of her best friends. Nevertheless, Ida Mae recalled, "While we were going to church, the mother told me that the boy was having problems with some of his classmates and a professor at school; also, he was not making good grades and some students were giving him a hard time." She also recalled that the mother tried to work out the situation so that Ronald would improve at school, which means that she was putting some pressure on the boy. She also used some negative reinforcement such as grounding the boy for a time and cutting off some privileges that he had had in the past. Consequently, Ronald may have concluded that it was still worthwhile to continue with the tricks in order to avoid school and the stress it was causing in his life.

According to the story, three days later, after the death of his Aunt, a new phenomenon began to manifest, a mysterious sound in Ronald's bedroom, as if "squeaking shoes were walking along his bed."[12] The noises could be heard only by Ronald. It is important to note that the squeaking shoe sounds were produced in his room and while he was out of the sight of any other family member. The family initially took the word of the boy for granted, and did not further question him or the account. However, after six days of squeaking shoes, the mother and the grandmother decided to go into his room and lie down with him on the bed to verify if the sound would be produced in their presence.

After a few minutes, they all heard the sound of moving feet, but this time they seemed to be marching towards them. They all suspected that the sounds might be connected to the death of Aunt Dorothy, who, they believed, might have been trying to communicate with them. The mother then asked: "Is this you, Aunt Dorothy?" There was no response, so the mother continued thus: "If you are Aunt Dorothy, knock three times." Then there were waves of air striking the faces of the grandmother, the mother, and the boy, after which three distinct knocks were heard (J.R., p. 1).

This story relates the presence of the mother, the grandmother, and the boy as the main characters. However, where is the father throughout this episode? He appears to be out of the picture. Could it be, as we have hypothesized, that he was hidden somewhere, conveying the message via the knocks to convince his superstitious wife to allow their son to go to St. Louis? The wife was already convinced that the knocks were related to the death of Aunt Dorothy. Regarding the air that struck their faces, we do not necessarily have to attribute it to a supernatural explanation: when doors or windows are open on a windy day, bursts of air may move around the house randomly.

The story also relates that, when the mother and the grandmother did not pay attention to the scratching sound of the bed, it would start to shake like a bed in a hotel with a shaking mechanism. Again, as preposterous as this explanation may sound, we have to consider that the father as a skilled electrician may have created the mechanism or device through which the bed could move; all Ronald needed to know was where such a button or starting mechanism was located. Indeed, the button may have been near the bed, so that Ronald could easily reach it at such time when his mother and grandmother were not paying close attention to him. Given the surprise factor, it would not have been difficult for Ronald to deceive his relatives in their altered mental states.

The story continues with the manifestation of still another phenomenon, such as when the coverlet of the bed was pulled out from under the mattress and its edges stood up above the bed's surface in a curled form as though held up with starch. When a bystander touched the bedspread, the sides fell back to a normal position. This may appear as a paranormal phenomenon, but how many times have we have seen this trick performed by a magician on television, where pieces of bedspread have been manipulated to appear as if they were held up by starch and then touched until they fell back to a normal position? A magician's basic manual may easily explain this trick. A simple mechanical device might cause the same effect by rigging the bedspread. Ronald's father had the technical knowledge to create such a device.

In a subtle way, the mother got the message that the spirits were trying to convey. However, still not completely convinced, she was reluctant to allow her son to go to St. Louis. The father, however, proposed that such a trip might actually bring the ordeal to an end. His idea was that, if they all traveled to St. Louis, the phenomena could be left behind in Maryland and might even stop.

Interestingly, to allay any remaining doubt during the discussion, Ronald needed something even more dramatic to close the deal. Thus "Go to St. Louis," a new, instant, dramatic mark, appeared on his body. As the Jesuit Report relates: "On one evening the word 'Louis'[13] was written on the boy's ribs in deep red. Next when there was some question of the time of departure, the word 'Saturday' was written plainly on the boy's hip."[14]

Concerning the marks, it is important to note that most of the time they appeared when he was out of the sight of his family—moreover, in a place where sharp objects were kept. What an interesting scenario! It obviously made it possible for him to create the conditions for self-inflicted marks, if necessary, in order to convince the reluctant mother. Could it be that he made the marks on himself? There is a high possibility that it may have been so. Moreover, according to Allen, the mother saw marks that spelled out in blood the single word "Louis." What did she actually see? Allen's description of the event gives us this response: "When questions of departure were discussed … Robbie doubled up in pain and let out a moan. He pulled on his pajamas. On his hip his mother saw blood ooze through his skin. It was as if scratches were emerging from him, as if something were cleaving at him from inside. The glistening scratches formed the word 'Saturday.'"[15]

This description tells us what the mother actually saw, namely, "blood oozing through the skin." It appears that she was looking at marks from which blood emerged after a cut had been made; in other words, this did not appear to be an instantaneous phenomenon. A pathologist consulted on the case has indicated that blood oozes as if emerging from the inside when a cut has been produced by a sharp object. The aforementioned description of the marks suggests what appear to be opening cuts from which blood emerged. Can we actually read words that appear after blood has emerged and the words are covered by blood? In response to this question, the dermatologist stated: "What seems more astonishing is the nature of the marks and circumstances in which they take place. The entire agenda of a trip is presented via the marks with astonishing precision; even though the marks may have been altered by the phenomenon, they can be very clearly read in terms of the destination, day of departure, and the length of time" (Fierro, 1997).[16]

Can we read bleeding marks? The dermatologist's comment contradicts Allen's version. Might the marks actually be rashes? Schulze provides a very interesting description of them. Contrary to what Allen led us to believe, in his description of the marks he stated that he saw scratches that were not readable and appeared to be marks, such as a rash (letter, dated March 25, 1949).

It is important to realize that marks produced by a sharp object differ from those produced by fingernails. Furthermore, the spirit possessing Ronald continues to lay down exact details of the proposed trip to St. Louis. When the question of the length of time for the stay in St. Louis is raised, the marks answer in blood: 3½ weeks. I wonder how somebody can read a mark that indicates in numbers and in blood such a clear message. Again, Dr. Jorge Fierro, the dermatologist consulted on the case, indicated that even if the marks had been caused by a sharp object, they would have to be very big and clear to be readable. Also, rashes are more likely to be caused by fingernails when we scratch our skin. The later explanation seems to be a more plausible explanation for the marks that appeared on Ronald's body.

Like a travel agent scheduling a trip, the spirit indicates a reasonable period of time for a vacation. One has to ask, if a spirit was possessing Ronald, why would it be interested in such details as going to St. Louis on a Saturday for three weeks and a half? Why didn't the entity choose a place such as Disneyland or some other location in the country? Why precisely to St. Louis where the preferred aunt lived? Why were all the marks rejecting the uncomfortable idea of going to school? We can understand that a diabolical entity may reject sacred places, but hardly a school precisely. The Roman Ritual indicates that one of the signs of possession is that a diabolical entity rejects sacred objects, but never in the history of exorcism and possession has such as entity rejected non-religious objects such as a school.

The Jesuit Report, in its account of the family's discussion of the possibility of sending Ronald to school while in St. Louis, relates: "There was some question of sending R. to school during his visit here, but the message, 'No,' appeared on his wrists; also a large 'n' on both legs. The mother feared disobeying this order" (J.R., p. 2). The mother said later that she was compelled to obey the messages and stopped discussing the issue of schooling with Ronald, afraid that he would suffer because of the marks that were making her son bleed.

Finally, after a long ordeal to convince the mother, she conceded; the entity suffering from school phobia accomplished its goal. The mother needed a long time to be persuaded, which had now had been done very efficiently by all these events, apparently caused by the possessing entity.

There are certain characteristics of the case that support the hypothesis that the boy inflicted the marks on himself. The "smoking gun" of the initial phenomenon was the Reverend Schulze, the Lutheran minister who initially became involved in the case. When the family took him to see their child, he examined the marks that had appeared on the body of the boy; this is the way he described them: "[B]ut meantime, words appeared on the boy's body, according to the family and friends. My physician and I saw no words, but we did see nerve reactions to rashes which had the appearance of scratches. However, according to the family report on this event the rashes looked more like words, indicating that the boy had to be taken to St. Louis" (J.R., p. 2).

From the above passage we can infer that the marks evidently did not look like words, as the family had determined; they just looked like superficial scratches similar to nerve reactions –marks that, if done by the boy on himself, would not have been dangerous or indicate serious damage (like the person who apparently wants to commit suicide but really just wants to call attention to himself without doing serious damage). These superficial marks might actually have been, as Schulze's medical doctor indicated, nerve rashes. We see how Schulze—in spite of being a minister—was not a credulous person, but actually tried to include a scientific perspective by inviting his own medical doctor to examine the child.

There is yet another possibility, namely, that some of the marks might have been real, but the result of stress affecting the skin, not produced by a spirit. It is important to note that one of the most sensitive body parts to be affected by stress is the skin. We have, in this case, a psychological stress scenario that may have led the boy to such nerve reactions. For instance, he had been under a lot of stress because of the schooling situation, as Ida Mae pointed out: "The mother told me that Ronald was having problems with his grades at school and that she was pressuring him to improve his performance" (notes from Ida Mae interview, 1990).

Dermatologists know well the effects of stress on the skin, as Lachman[17] has pointed out. "A number of common reactions to emotional stimulus have been specified. These include ... reddening or flushing of the skin surface.... A pattern of roughness in the skin consisting of multiple swellings or protuberances...." He further adds, "The psychogenic nature of various skin disorders is attested to by the following pattern: Rashes may break out in emotional situations or response to frustration" (p. 117).

Another possibility is a condition known in the DSM-IV as conversion reaction or hysteria. Again, Jorge Fierro, a dermatologist consulted for the case, indicated that during this condition the skin becomes so sensitive that a sharp object or even fingernails lightly drawn over its surface can immediately raise welts. Could it be that Ronald was suffering from such a conversion reaction that facilitated the making of the marks on his skin? It is important to recall that the marks were mostly produced when he was out of the sight of his family or when he suddenly and deliberately opened some part of his clothing to show new ones. It seems plausible that the marks were already there. They never appeared spontaneously, at least in the initial stages of the ordeal.

In sum, is it possible to conclude that circumstances surrounding the case might lead us to speculate that the fraud and tricks hypothesis is a partial viable explanation in the case of the Mount Rainier Exorcism? The answer is affirmative; clearly, at least serious reservations and doubts can be attached to this case. What follows is a summary of several reasons that lead us to the aforementioned conclusion.

- A motive to proceed in a fraudulent way: An adolescent under stress and a lot of pressure from his mother to improve in school, who wanted to go to live in St. Louis with his favorite aunt and thus avoid going to school.
- A father who wanted by all means to please his son but without openly confronting his credulous but domineering wife. Moreover, he had the technical knowledge to manufacture a few tricks to convince his reluctant wife and obtain her consent.
- A superstitious wife who was open to obeying a message from the spirits. It is important to indicate, in this regard, that she was a firm believer in spiritualistic practices. She had participated in mediumistic practices along with all other family members. Moreover, there was the manifestation of another phenomenon, in which a table in the kitchen turned over without any action on the boy's part, milk and food moved off the table, and the like, in which there appeared to be no intention or influence from the boy. Nevertheless, some of these phenomena may be explained also by the fraud hypothesis, although not here.

It is, however, important to remark that the fraud hypothesis cannot by itself explain all the phenomena in this case, such as the spontaneous marks that later appeared on the boy before several witnesses—particularly those that appeared on his body during the exorcism that took place in St. Louis at the Alexian Brothers Hospital. In this particular event, the witnesses are much more reliable than the parents, as they included priests and probably some mental health professionals or medical doctors, who may well have participated in the process before the exorcism resumed, even though we have so far no actual records of such participation. Marks spontaneously appeared on the boy while many people were looking at him, and it is hard to imagine that all the participants were deceived by him. Also, assuming that the diary found in the Alexian Brothers Hospital constitutes a reliable source of information on the case, then we have a phenomenon that cannot easily be explained away by the fraud hypothesis. Therefore, following the model proposed by Father Nicola, we will proceed with the second hypothesis in the hierarchy, which may provide a more suitable explanation until we can find moral certainty.

12

The "Occam's Razor Principle" and the Natural Scientific Hypothesis (Especially Psychological)

For many centuries, in various parts of the world, mental illness was considered the result of demonic possession. We may recall the incident in Gadarene, an ancient city of the Middle East southeast of the Sea of Galilee, described in the Bible as the place where Jesus cast demons out of a man and into a herd of swine, which then threw themselves into the sea (Matthew 8:28–34). This is an example of exorcism being used as a form of treatment. It was not until the end of the 19th century that scientific accounts of this type of mental phenomenon began to be accepted as viable explanations of ostensible cases of demonic possession. However, before considering any psychological descriptions of the case of Ronald in the Mount Rainier Exorcism, we will examine the psychological profile of Ronald as it stood before the supposed possession took place. This profile will provide us with a more complete picture of his mental state prior to the ordeal, along with some psychological clues that may have led to the "possession case."

According to the Lutheran minister Luther Schulze, the adolescent, when the initial phenomena began to appear, was initially evaluated by the family's physician. The doctor placed the boy in the hands of the local mental hygiene clinic, where he was treated by Dr. Mabel Rose, a physician at the University of Maryland. She held two interviews with the boy there and also ran a complete physical check-up of his condition.[1]

According to the medical records on the case, he was found to be a normal boy, albeit somewhat high-strung. A psychiatrist who was also consulted in the case reported that he did not believe that the phenomena surrounding the adolescent were real, reporting that, in his opinion, the boy "was quite normal." Moreover, when the family's physician went to see the boy at the clinic, he recommended that he be treated with barbital (a long-acting barbiturate that depresses most metabolic processes at high doses; used as a hypnotic or sedative, it may induce dependence).[2]

Interestingly, staff members at the clinic, rather than showing great concern for the boy's condition, which they found to be normal, were more worried about the reputation of the clinic, which was treating a case "considered, by some, to be a demonic possession case." Judging that this situation could bring a negative reputation to a hitherto respectable medical institution, they hoped that news of the case would not be spread outside the clinic.[3]

This situation was discussed by Richard Darnell, Director of the Society of Parapsychology in Washington, D.C., in 1949, via numerous correspondence exchanges with Dr. J.B. Rhine, a member of the Society. Darnell, who had been involved in the case by establishing contact with the Reverend Schulze via the Washington Society for Parapsychology, had talked to both the medical doctors and the psychiatrist who had evaluated Ronald. According to Darnell, even though both doctors had determined that Ronald was a normal boy, they nevertheless thought that there was "something unusual about this case," although they did not further expand on the issue.[4]

Based on the above, we might assume that, in addition to the physical tests, a psychiatric evaluation by the psychiatrist, Dr. Ullman, who conducted the second evaluation of Ronald, may have been followed by a series of mental tests, perhaps including a personality assessment such as the Rorschach Test in order to detect any sign of psychopathology. Evidently, if there had been any psychological disturbance, it could have had been detected by the psychiatrist. Nevertheless, he rendered a diagnosis of normality.

Since this is just speculation on the procedures that the psychiatrist may have followed, it is also possible that the psychiatrist may have just clinically interviewed the adolescent and the family to make his diagnosis. We have only the sketchy information on the case included in the letters from the Society of Parapsychology in Washington led by Richard Darnell.

Moreover, is important to note that, at this stage, Ronald presented a profile of a normal young adolescent, according to the reports presented by Richard Darnell to Dr. Rhine. Furthermore, another interesting dimension of the case is that the problem Ronald was facing was not considered to be very serious from either a religious or a medical standpoint. We must recall that the Reverend Schulze's medical doctor also evaluated Ronald in order to determine the nature of the marks that appeared on the boy's body, concluding that they seemed to be nervous rashes rather than actual marks.

The psychological reactions of the parents, at this point, were of skepticism regarding the medical opinions that "did not seem to fit their expectations on the case." They were convinced that it was a case of demonic possession; thus the opinions of the experts were clearly off the mark for them. Acting on their own convictions, they put aside the opinions of the Reverend Schulze and the medical doctors in order to seek the opinion of a spiritualist. At this point Schulze confronted the spiritualist with his own skepticism, as he replicated the trick the spiritualist had performed before the family of the boy in order to convince them of her powers.[5] This issue will be addressed later.

To sum up, regarding Ronald's psychological state of mind, the medical records at the time of the initial evaluations found that he was a normal boy, somewhat high-strung, but with no psychopathology detected. It seems, then, that the medical evaluations, which may or may not have included psychological tests and an EEG, found nothing wrong with Ronald.

We can add to these preliminary medical and psychological evaluations, information about the personality of the boy, offered by close friends of the family, who indicated that he was an introvert but showed no signs of psychopathology. It is unfortunate, of course, that no medical records of the time have ever been found or revealed that might provide us with a more complete picture of his personality. Regarding the psychological dynamics of the family, they do not seem to indicate a very serious high level of stress or a conflictive profile that could have affected the adolescent in a negative way. For example, Ida Mae, a personal assistant to the Reverend Schulze, a friend of the family, indicated in a personal interview with me that the parents were a normal couple with no more than the usual discussions and differences. According to her, they were good workers, regular churchgoers, and very friendly and social. Their relationship with their only son also seemed to be smooth. Of course, while Ronald's family appeared to be normal on the outside, we can hardly have access to what actually happened when they were alone.

Regarding the marks that spontaneously branded the boy's body, it is important to note that there is a disorder known as "conversion disorder" (American Psychiatric Association, DSM-IV, 1994)[6] that may have caused the marks (although one cannot easily explain the actual mechanism for such phenomena). According to the DSM-IV: "Traditionally, the term conversion derives from the hypothesis that the individual's somatic symptoms represent a symbolic resolution of an unconscious psychological conflict, reducing anxiety and serving to keep the conflict out of awareness ('primary gain'). The individual may also derive 'secondary gain' from the conversion symptoms— that is, external benefits are obtained or noxious duties and responsibilities are evaded" (p. 453).

In support of the aforementioned diagnosis, there is a diagnostic criterion established by the DSM-IV that leads us to the conclusion that the 14-year-old adolescent may have suffered from a condition known as Conversion Reaction. For instance, he was undergoing "serious psychological turmoil and conflict" as a result of his unhappiness at school, where he was clashing with other students. Moreover, he was facing a conflictive situation with his mother, who ignored his problems at school and was pressuring him to attend classes regularly. This conflict may well have been causing him to experience considerable distress. Moreover, this stress, in turn, may have resulted in a psychosomatic disorder that affected his skin, causing a rash reaction. It is important to note that a connection between an emotional stimulus and certain specific skin problems has been established. As pointed out by Lachman (1972)[7]: "A number of common reactions to emotional stimulus have been specified. These include ... reddening or flushing of the skin surface ... [such as] a pattern of roughness in the skin consisting of multiple swellings and protuberances" (p. 117). Lachman adds that the psychogenic nature of various skin disorders, such as rashes, may break out in emotional situations or in response to frustration (p. 118), among them the aforementioned psychological condition that may create such skin reactions is "conversion reaction," or what used to be called "hysteria." According to a dermatologist consulted on the case (Fierro, 2006),[8] "in some cases of conversion reaction, the skin becomes so sensitive that fingernails lightly drawn over its surface immediately raise red welts." Indeed, that Ronald was suffering from a skin disorder caused by the deep stress he was undergoing, has been confirmed by one of the letters addressed by the Reverend Schulze to Dr. J.B. Rhine, indicating that, when Schulze and his personal physician saw the alleged "St. Louis marks" on the boy's body, they "looked more like those caused by nerve reactions."[9] If the diagnosis of conversion reaction is correct in the case of Ronald, his psychological condition would have had to meet the criteria established by the DSM-IV for this somatoform disorder. Its main feature is an alteration or loss of physical functioning that suggests a physical disorder, but is instead the expression of a psychological conflict or need. Conversion reaction is a neurotic disorder characterized by development of an illness. Typical symptoms include a loss or alteration of a sensory or motor functioning (deafness, blindness, or paralysis) (DSM-IV, 1994). The condition, according to Lachman (1972),[10] is usually temporary, and the symptoms appear to resolve a problem for the individual, at least temporarily (p. 15).

For instance, explains Lachman, an individual may develop conversion reaction blindness in order to resign from a particular job or to avoid an unpleasant situation. The symptoms relate to the motives and conflicts of the persons who display them (Lachman, 1972).[11] The classic symptoms of the disorder, according to the DSM-IV, are those that suggest neurological diseases such as paralysis, aphoria, seizures, akinesia, dyskinesia, blindness, etc.

Two mechanisms have been suggested by the DSM-IV to explain what "benefits" the person derives from having conversion symptoms. In the first mechanism, the person achieves "primary gain" by keeping an internal conflict or need out of awareness. In such cases there is a temporal relationship between an environmental stimulus that is apparently related to a psychological conflict or need and the initiation or exacerbation of the symptom. For example, after an argument, inner conflict about the expression of rage may be expressed as "aphoria" or as "paralysis" of the arm; in such cases, the symptom, explains the DSM -IV, has a symbolic meaning that is a representation and partial solution of the underlying psychological conflict.

Regarding the second mechanism, the person achieves "secondary gain" by avoiding a particular activity that is noxious to him or her and getting support from the environment that otherwise might not be forthcoming. For instance, with a paralyzed hand, a soldier can avoid firing a gun. Moreover, explains Lachman, an individual may develop conversion blindness or deafness to get out of a particular job or avoid an unpleasant or painful situation.

Moreover, in explaining the convulsions suffered by the boy, Lachman (1972)[12] cited Kutash, an expert on conversion disorders, who, while "commenting on the convulsions produced sometimes during conversion reaction," stated: "Occasionally in some cases of conversion reaction, one sees cases of hysterical convulsions or fits resembling epileptic seizures but distinguishable from them by the fact that the patient does not usually bite his tongue, injure himself or suffer incontinence. His pupillary reflex to light remains unaffected. The convulsions in the hysteric usually occur in the presence of other people" (p. 19).

In summing up the comments of the aforementioned medical authorities, in the context of my assessment of the case, one may ask: Was the Mount Rainier boy suffering from conversion reaction and coprolalia (the excessive and uncontrollable use of foul or obscene language) that were later aggravated by the exorcism? I suspect that the answer could be affirmative in this case. It is important to note that, if one proffers a diagnosis of conversion reaction, one is assuming that the symptoms were real, that the documents were truthful, and that the boy was not malingering (that is, manufacturing all those things to attract attention, avoid going to school, and get a trip to St. Louis to visit his favorite aunt, thereby obtaining multiple benefits). But one must recognize that I am only speculating and that my diagnosis may be questioned. And yet, in correspondence addressed by the Reverend Schulze to Rhine in 1949, Schulze confirms the existence of the marks in a way that further supports my proposed diagnosis. In this regard, he points out: "[W]ords appeared on the boy, according to the family and friends. My physician and I saw no words, but we did see nerve reaction rashes which had the appearance of scratches."[13]

Moreover, according to Schulze, in regard to the convulsions suffered by the boy, the family's physician insisted that they treat him with barbital[14] to stop the convulsions. Also, in another letter addressed to Rhine, he mentioned the use of barbital to treat Ronald. Of course, the prescription of this drug is not conclusive evidence in opposition to or in favor of my diagnosis.

In addition to the symptoms mentioned above, which support the conversion reaction diagnosis, there is another element in the case that supports such a diagnosis from a psychological standpoint. As we have previously mentioned, the family dynamics had created for the boy a very stressful situation. He was having some difficulties at school, and his parents, particularly his mother, were putting pressure on him to continue attending in spite of his psychological problems.

Consequently, the school had obviously, as I have indicated above, become a noxious stimulus for Ronald, which he was trying to avoid by all means. Such a stimulus, in turn, may have led to a stressful reaction and also have created what the DSM-IV calls a "psychological conflict or need" that evolved into a conversion disorder. The aforementioned speculation on the case is supported by the fact that different marks appeared on the boy's body, such as two large letter "N"s on his legs. Also, when the possibility of sending him to school while in St. Louis was raised by his mother, the marks expressed a complete rejection of the idea of attending school there.

The above situation, while far from conclusive, fits the second mechanism suggested by the DSM-IV to explain the benefits derived by the person suffering from the condition of having a conversion symptom. That is, the person achieves "secondary gain" by avoiding a particular activity that is noxious to him or her, and obtaining support from the environment that otherwise might not be forthcoming. In the particular case of the marks, they obviously helped Ronald attain his goals of avoiding school and going to live with his favorite aunt. For instance, when the mark "St. Louis" appeared on the boy's body, the mother exclaimed rapidly, "We'll go to St. Louis! We'll go to St. Louis." She explained later that she felt compelled to obey the messages (Allen, 1993).[15]

Another example of conversion reaction, similar to the case of Ronald, is the case of Mariana, a patient whom I saw in consultation at the hospital. She was sent to treatment by her otorhinolaryngologist, because she was experiencing, very intensely, the smell of human feces in her place of employment. The smell was so strong that she could not stand being in her job more than one hour at a time. The supervisors checked for the origin of this terrible smell but found none, nor did they experience the same smell as Mariana did. She insisted on being seen by the company's physician, who referred her to an otorhinolaryngologist, who, after several physical tests, found nothing wrong from an organic perspective. He decided to send her for mental treatment, after discarding any organic cause except phantosmia (an olfactory hallucination wherein one detects smells that are not really present in the environment).

When she arrived at my office, she told me immediately that it smelled like human feces too. Since people had been fixing the toilet in the office, I responded, "You are not wrong … it really does smell like feces in here, but there is a reason." I asked under what specific circumstances she experienced this smell or if it was general in that she experienced the smell everywhere. She replied, "Just when I am at work or with my boss. I have not told him this … but he really stinks, particularly when he gets mad at me. I just run away from him and leave my job." Her comments provided me with a clue that there was something wrong with her, so I asked if her boss was normally a clean and neat person. She replied positively. I asked then, "Does it happen generally when he gets on your case?" She replied, yes.

I realized that her boss represented a noxious stimulus to her, and her mind was creating that smell in him. At that point she would ask for permission to leave her job, which was her secondary gain by avoiding this person in a position of authority who was frequently tough on her. Once I recommended that she be restationed in an area apart from where she had been working with her boss, the smell immediately disappeared. We know that there are organic causes (a subjacent tumor, neurological disorders, convulsions, Parkinson's disease, and others) to account for this phantom smell; however, when there is an underlying physical cause, this is a chronic condition that is manifested in many places and under very different circumstances. In this case, Mariana hated her boss and wanted to be removed from his area of influence. Once this happened, she was "cured."

13

Psychic Detectives
The Parapsychological Hypothesis

Parapsychologists have longtime investigated poltergeist phenomena as a possible explanation for the phenomena surrounding demonic possession cases. In folklore and parapsychology, a poltergeist (German for "noisy ghost") is a type of ghost or other supernatural being supposedly responsible for physical disturbances, such as loud noises and objects being moved or destroyed around the poltergeist subject. Most accounts of poltergeists describe movement or levitation of objects, such as furniture and cutlery, or noises such as knocking on doors. Poltergeists are purportedly capable of pinching, biting, hitting and tripping people.

Some researchers have proposed explanatory models to explain the poltergeist phenomena. Many claimed poltergeist events have proved on investigation to be pranks.[1] Skeptic Joe Nickell says that claimed poltergeist incidents typically originate from "an individual who is motivated to cause mischief." According to Nickell: "In the typical poltergeist outbreak, small objects are hurled through the air by unseen forces, furniture is overturned, or other disturbances occur—usually just what could be accomplished by a juvenile trickster determined to plague credulous adults."[2]

> Time and again in other "poltergeist" outbreaks, witnesses have reported an object leaping from its resting place supposedly on its own, when it is likely that the perpetrator had secretly obtained the object sometime earlier and waited for an opportunity to fling it, even from outside the room—thus supposedly proving he or she was innocent.[3]

Others, such as Lange and Houran (1998),[4] indicate that research in anomalistic psychology could explain poltergeist activity by psychological factors such as illusion, memory lapses and wishful thinking. In a study conducted by Lange and Houran in 1998, in their conclusions they wrote that poltergeist experiences are delusions "resulting from the affective and cognitive dynamics of percipients' interpretation of ambiguous stimuli."

Also, Nandor Fodor,[5] who was at one time Sigmund Freud's associate, pioneered the theory that poltergeists are external manifestations of conflicts within the subconscious mind rather than autonomous entities with minds of their own. He proposed that poltergeist disturbances are caused by human agents suffering from some form of emotional stress or tension and compared reports of poltergeist activity to hysterical conversion symptoms resulting from emotional tension of the subject.

Moreover, William Roll (1972)[6] hypothesized that poltergeist activity can be explained by psychokinesis, the movement of objects at a distance using the mind. Furthermore, poltergeist activity has often been believed to be the work of malicious spirits. According to Allan Kardec, the founder of spiritism, poltergeists are manifestations of disembodied spirits of low level, belonging to the sixth class of the third order. They are believed to be closely associated with the elements (fire, air, water, earth).[7] For the Catholic Church, the poltergeist phenomena are the result of the demonic entity possessing the victim of the poltergeist activity. In this regard, Scott Rogo, in his fine study *The Poltergeist Experience*, carefully developed the theory that possession cases are examples of the operation of an agency which is part of the victim's own psyche, but which has attained a kind of independence of its own, and is thus the cause of the strange phenomena. Framed in the above context, the Mount Rainier case will be next evaluated to find out if it fits any of the above explanatory hypotheses, particularly the poltergeist hypothesis via the psychokinesis theory held by William Roll.

News about the Mt. Rainier case reached J.B. and Louisa Rhine in 1949 through the young minister, Luther Miles Schulze, to whom the parents of Ronald had appealed for help. In response, Schulze, who was the family's minister and friend, became involved in the case. From the boy's family, Schulze learned about the strange phenomena surrounding him such as levitation of objects, dishes toppled from tables, and weird voices. To Schulze, interested as he was in parapsychology and familiar with the work of J.B. Rhine at the Parapsychology Laboratory at Duke University, the phenomena reported to him seemed similar to those manifested in conventional poltergeist cases, but he nonetheless took a skeptical position. This stance led him to ask the family for permission to take the boy to his own premises, in order to confirm the phenomena they had reported to him. As Father John Nicola, an expert on demonic possession and exorcism, stated in his book *Diabolical Possession and Exorcism*[8] regarding Schulze's position:

> Therefore, he took the boy one night to his premises and observed him closely before going to sleep in order to determine if the phenomena told to him were real or if the boy was faking it. It turned out that the events that took place that night completely shook his skepticism and led him to believe that he was dealing with genuine phenomena that could not be explained by fraud. The phenomena appeared

to him more of a poltergeist nature, so he decided to contact Dr. J.B. Rhine at Duke University in order to find a viable explanation of what he had witnessed. He had read about the work of J.B. Rhine at Duke and this seemed to be the best way to proceed with the case (p. 10).

Thus in a letter[9] dated March 21, 1949, addressed to Dr. J.B. Rhine at the Parapsychology Laboratory at Duke University, he wrote as follows:

> We have in our congregation a family who is being disturbed by poltergeist phenomena.... I had him in my home for the nights of February 17–19 to observe him by myself. Chairs moved with him, and one threw him out. His bed shook whenever he was on it. When he was in bed with me, mine vibrated. There was no apparent motion of his body. I then made a bed on the floor for him and this glided over the floor.... Would you or someone else from your staff be interested in studying the case?

From the minister's description, Dr. Rhine felt it sounded like a poltergeist attack (Brian, 1982).[10] Therefore, in reply to his request for help, Rhine offered a preliminary explanation of the phenomena that were leading the boy to believe that he was the victim of mysterious forces.

At the same time, he acknowledged that some of the phenomena were not exactly of that nature. In his reply to the Reverend Schulze, in a letter[11] dated April 2, 1949, he declared: "As you know, the most likely explanation is that the boy is, himself, led to create the effect of being the victim of mysterious forces and might be sincerely convinced of it. Such movements as those of the chair and the bed might, from your brief account of them, have originated within himself." Moreover, he questioned Schulze about the conditions under which he had observed the phenomena in order to check that he was not deceived by such deficient environmental surroundings such as poor lighting and the like. He also wished to determine if he might actually be relying on the account of the boy. Thus he wrote, "I presume you observed the movement in good light and were not in any way relying upon his account of it."[12]

Furthermore, Rhine expressed interest in investigating the case himself, to see if the phenomena would occur in his presence as well, thereby convincing him of their parapsychological character. Late in the case, Dr. Rhine assumed an even more guarded position, suggesting the possibility of trickery on the part of the adolescent. Thus in a subsequent letter[13] (dated April 21, 1949), he asked Schulze for a firsthand report of the phenomena that he had witnessed: "Could you give an account of the firsthand evidence you have of the phenomena—what you actually saw the boy do and witnessed in his presence? If you could be entirely sure that the phenomena are not explained by trickery conscious or unconscious.... The reason I take a guarded position is that a number of these cases have been reduced to clever trickery, and since we are not ordinarily prepared for the unusual (rather, pathological) sort of faking that is sometimes practiced, we are not as guarded as would be required to see everything that is going on."

In response to Rhine's request, Schulze prepared a report on Ronald's case and gave it to him, Dr. Rhine carefully reviewed the report, asking Schulze for further clarification on some details that he had previously presented. Rhine felt that the written version seemed to contain some information that Schulze had not reported orally, but the discrepancies were satisfactorily cleared up. In his next letter, Dr. Rhine declared: "There were a few details in your oral account that I had not found in your written report.... Was the light on in the room? Where were you located when the chair was overturned? ... Would you mind telling me what your emotions were, if you can remember?"

The Reverend Schulze replied to the above questions in the same letter, with notations at the side of the questions. Regarding the light being on, he replied "Yes"; regarding the chair being overturned, he replied, "I was standing in front when it toppled.... I wanted to see if it really would go over" (letter dated July 1, 1949).[14]

It is important to note that, up to this point in the case, the Reverend Schulze had followed Rhine's advice to look at the phenomena carefully and from a guarded position. Not only had he consulted J.B. Rhine, with whose work he was familiar, but he had also presented the case to the Society of Parapsychology in Washington, D.C. Interestingly, he first hypothesized that the phenomena surrounding the case were due to clever trickery by the adolescent. Later, when he witnessed actual phenomena that he could not explain by normal means, he moved on to the hypothesis that some sort of psychological or medical mechanism might be required to explain what was happening. Therefore, he took the boy to his personal physician for a medical evaluation and persuaded the family to take him to the Mental Hygiene Clinic of Maryland, where a diagnosis of normality was subsequently rendered.

It was only after having followed these scientific procedures that he decided to contact Dr. Rhine in order to determine if a parapsychological mechanism might account for the happenings. Furthermore, despite his religious background, he never proposed a supernatural explanation of the case. Instead, he went through the scientific model of the hierarchy of causality proposed by John Nicola to explain cases of demonic possession. It was this scientific attitude that eventually led the family to release him from the case.

For instance, in explaining the marks that had appeared on the boy's body, which had been evaluated by him and his physician, he provided a natural explanation for them. In a letter dated March 21, 1949, he wrote: "[B]ut meantime, words appeared on the boy's body, according to the family and friends. My physician and I saw no words, but we did see some nerve reaction rashes which had the appearance of scratches."

As it can be seen, the Reverend Schulze questioned the nature of the marks to the extent of having his own physician evaluate them in order to determine what they were. Furthermore, he tried to maintain a distance from the family's reports, using such phrases as "according to the family and friends," or "they tell me." That is, he never appears as a credulous believer of what was reported to him. His tone throughout the entire ordeal seems to be coming from somebody who was rather critical of what was being told to him. Moreover, at one point, he cautioned the family about being too credulous of the account of the exorcism told to them by the priest involved, to the point where he even suggested therapy for the family (letter dated April 19, 1949).[15]

It should be noted that the Reverend Schulze's critical attitude was the opposite of that taken by Father William Bowdern, one of the priests involved in the exorcism. He and another priest who rendered the diagnosis of possession were very accepting of the family's accounts, which they, in turn, used to make their diagnosis of demonic possession. Indeed, they proceeded with an exorcism even though they had not studied the case as extensively as the Roman Ritual recommends. In sum, the Lutheran minister took a guarded position, first considering the hypothesis that the case could be fraudulent, and then moving on to the next level to try to explain the phenomena by medical and psychological means. It was only after all that, when he realized that he himself was witnessing phenomena that he could not explain scientifically, that he moved on to the hypothesis that the phenomena might have been caused by poltergeist-like activity.

It is important to note that the aforementioned critical and scientific attitude assumed by the Reverend Schulze was applauded by Dr. J.B. Rhine, who wrote in this regard: "It seems to me that you did everything that an intelligent, capable minister could have done under the circumstances, and I am greatly impressed by the real service you gave to the family. This is true ministry" (letter dated July 1, 1949).[16] It could even be said that the Reverend Schulze, perhaps unconsciously, embraced the principle of scientific economy, which states that "when a natural and ordinary explanation is possible, we do not have to resort to unusual and extraordinary causes even though the potentiality, and the possibility, are always there."[17] In other words, we are not to look for preternatural explanations unless we have previously demonstrated the impossibility of a natural explanation.

In the sequence of events, the Reverend Schulze tried to minimize the phenomena that had been witnessed by the family. In order to prove that the events "were a figment of their imagination," he took the boy to his premises and told the family, "I assure you that nothing of what you said about the phenomena is going to take place in my house."[18]

As he later related, "I took the boy to my premises for a night and decided to sleep in the same room with him to witness by myself the supposed phenomena. I carefully observed to see if anything strange would happen around the boy."

However, what he witnessed next that night "shook his critical and skeptical attitude." As he related in the interview, "the bed of the boy began to shake whenever he was on it, and more astonishing, the reverend's bed also vibrated when the boy was in the bed with him."[19]

He also recalled, "the bed vibrated like one of those motel vibrator beds, but much faster." Then, as he related in a letter to J.B. Rhine, "There was no apparent motion of his body [when the bed vibrated] and his hands were at a standstill" (letter dated March 21, 1949). Moreover, that same night, a heavy chair in which he had placed the boy moved with him and threw him out. When he was questioned by Rhine regarding where he was when the chair was overturned, he answered, "Standing in front when it toppled" (letter dated July 1, 1949).

For a skeptical man such as Schulze, the phenomena he witnessed that night must have been really astonishing and the experience even traumatic. Nevertheless, despite what he saw, he still did not accept the idea of a supernatural agency as the explanation. At this stage of the case, the family became impatient with his skeptical attitude and decided to return to the Catholic Church for help. That was when they moved to St. Louis, where the case fell into the hands of the Jesuits, who, in turn, performed an exorcism to free Ronald of his demons. This meant that J.B. Rhine could not personally investigate the case. However, he did visit the Reverend Schulze in D.C. in order to examine personally the place where the phenomena had happened in front of the minister.

Subsequently, Schulze had the opportunity to get his hands on the so-called Jesuit Report on the case, which was a detailed account of the exorcism performed on the adolescent in St. Louis. He also had access to the medical documents and reports on the case.

Up to this time, the Reverend Schulze maintained his critical position on the case and never suggested the idea of a supernatural agency in order to explain the phenomena.[20] He asserted that initially he believed the boy had faked some of the phenomena in order to accomplish his goal to go live in St. Louis with his favorite aunt. However, as the case evolved, he became convinced that there was something genuine in the phenomena surrounding the boy that he could not explain. As he recalled: "The boy was not faking it. I wondered if I was going screwy."[21] At the same time, he continued to seek a natural explanation or a parapsychological explanation, possibly in the form of a poltergeist case permeated with religious elements.

Indeed, one of the facets of the case that provided some sort of a hint that this was not a case of demonic possession was the lack of a feeling of a "diabolical presence." The Reverend Schulze insisted that he did not experience such a presence, which some experts claim is one of the characteristics of demonic possession (Martin, 1977).[22] When asked in a personal interview if he sensed or perceived the presence of some kind of demon the night that the boy spent at his premises, he replied with a firm no. Was the Reverend Schulze correct in his position that the Mt. Rainier case was that of a poltergeist and not one of demonic possession? This question is explored below, in the context of testimonies and events as reported by the boy's family.

The first step is to evaluate the reliability of the different testimonies and documents in order to learn if there are sufficient elements to render this case as one of poltergeists; this means paying particular attention to the Reverend Schulze's reports on the case, since he appears to be the most reliable witness because of his scientific and critical approach. In contrast, the Jesuits who performed the exorcism appeared to accept as credible the phenomena reported to them by the family, as they took them for granted as accurate. Moreover, before the actual exorcism, the Jesuits used the family reports for their diagnostic criteria, although they themselves had witnessed very few phenomena of a poltergeist nature that would have persuaded them to consider this an instance of demonic possession instead. They also failed to use the guarded position prescribed by the Rituale Romanum specifying a critical attitude and the necessity of looking at natural causes and psychological problems before diagnosing anything supernatural.

Furthermore, the family's testimony on the case must be considered cautiously, since there are elements therein that cast serious doubts on the veracity of their reports to the Jesuits—raising, in other words, the possibility of fraud, whether intentional or not. It is important to note at the start that they were very superstitious; at one point, they even called in a "spiritualist" to perform a healing ceremony. Therefore, their testimony may have been unintentionally biased from the start.

Regarding the spiritualist approach, the family decided to have a ritual known as the Powai in the initial stages of the ordeal, with the boy examined by a spiritual healer. It appears that the case began as an obsession about poltergeist activity, but ended up as demonic possession as a result of the decision to exorcise the boy. It is entirely possible that, if Ronald had never been exorcised, the Mt. Rainier case would never have developed into one of demonic possession.

At the same time, how do we explain the strange phenomena reported by the very skeptical Lutheran minister? Such activities often take place in the context of poorly controlled conditions, or are seen by witnesses who are misled by their altered perceptions of the events; in other words, if you are credulous, "you will call the devil and the devil will show up."[23]

The first element that appears to support the poltergeist hypothesis is the diagnosis provided by the psychiatrist who initially evaluated the boy. It comes to us through one of the letters written by the Reverend Schulze, who had permission from the family to examine the first medical report. Thus in a letter from Schulze to J.B. Rhine, he reports that Ronald was taken for a medical examination to the Mental Hygiene Clinic at the University of Maryland under the direction of Mabel Ross. In this letter he summarizes thus: "The report of the mental hygiene clinic ... indicates that the boy did not seem to want to grow up, but preferred holding onto his childhood" (letter, September 19, 1949).[24]

In response to Schulze's report of the doctor's diagnosis, J.B. Rhine replied, "The puberty hypothesis is the one to watch in this case" (letter September 21, 1949).[25] We can infer from Rhine's reply that he was using the words "puberty hypothesis" to refer to a poltergeist as an explanation of the phenomena. Some experts in poltergeist phenomena, such as Scott Rogo, have argued that the psychiatric and psychoanalytic interpretations of the case present us with an adolescent confronting a psychological conflict, which is a characteristic frequently found in a focal person or agent of a poltergeist phenomenon at the puberty or adolescence age. Consequently, the tension or stress produced by the psychological conflict could be released through subconscious psychokinesis, or PK (movement of physical objects by the mind without use of physical means).

In this regard, in the 1960s, William G. Roll, the project director of the Psychical Research Foundation in Durham, North Carolina, presented his theory and identified it as Recurrent Spontaneous Psychokinesis (RSPK). Roll researched reports of poltergeist occurrences over four centuries, which resulted in his belief that, most often, the "poltergeist" was an angry child or teenager who subconsciously caused the disturbances.[26]

The psychiatric diagnosis presents us with an adolescent undergoing a psychological conflict. What subsequently happened, however, was that Ronald reached adolescence through the ordeal of exorcism. The period of adolescence, which follows childhood, usually begins at age fourteen in men. It is typically characterized by rapid physical and mental development, often accompanied by emotional turmoil. Furthermore, being an adolescent means adapting to a different set of roles, values, and expectations. At this time, childlike games are left behind, as the adolescent is expected to assume new responsibilities with regard to education and family. The parents of adolescents expect them to behave according to a new set of adult roles and rules. At the same time, the new stage of life brings with it new privileges, which include being more independent. In sum, reaching adolescence not only implies fast physical and mental development, but also brings the assumption of different social roles, including meeting different expectations of how one spends one's time and energies.[27]

Consequently, the prospect of reaching adolescence, with its new roles and expectations, can be seen as threatening. Confronting the new stimuli and adapting to the new responsibilities may become very stressful for an adolescent who may not be willing to relinquish the privileges of childhood. According to Sigmund Freud, who saw adolescence as a time of crisis when inner impulses and outer requirements waged war with each other, leaving the adolescent caught in between.[28] It is in this context that we have the psychoanalytic diagnosis of the case indicating that "the child did not want to reach the next level of life which is adolescence and wanted to hold onto his childhood."[29]

In other words, growing up for Ronald may have meant sacrificing leisure time in exchange for more responsibilities than he was willing to assume. Therefore, he decided to hold onto his immaturity. These circumstances may have led Ronald into a psychological conflict that blocked his normal developmental process. As has been indicated by Erik Erikson, this is the stage of "Identity vs. Role Confusion. During this adolescent stage (age 12 to 18 years), the transition from childhood to adulthood is most important. Children are becoming more independent, and begin to look at the future in terms of career, relationships, families, housing, etc. The individual wants to belong to society."[30]

Also, according to Erikson, during this period, they explore possibilities and begin to form their own identity based upon the outcome of their explorations. Failure to establish a sense of identity within society ("I don't know what I want to be when I grow up") can lead to role confusion. Role confusion involves the individual's not being sure about himself or his place in society.

Moreover, in response to role confusion or identity crisis, an adolescent may begin to experiment with different lifestyles (e.g., work, education or political activities). Also, pressuring someone into an identity can result in rebellion in the form of establishing a negative identity, and in addition, a feeling of unhappiness.

Ronald's family, instead of encouraging the above process of healthy development, perhaps by engaging him in outside activities appropriate to his age group such as sports, pressed him to practice less social activities such as board games; his lack of interest in these games was reinforced by his Aunt Dorothy (called Harriet in Allen's book), who introduced him to the Ouija board as an alternate occupation (Allen, 1993). Indeed, "Aunt Harriet seems to have treated Robbie [that is, Ronald] more like a special friend than a nephew; she was a frequent visitor to the family and introduced him to the Ouija board" (p. 2). Moreover, Ronald, an only child, was particularly spoiled by his father, who wanted to please him in everything. It is, therefore, plausible that his father would support him even in activities that would contradict the interests and values of his wife. Consequently, there may have been conflict between his parents, with the mother pressuring the boy to comply with his responsibilities and attend school regularly.

Furthermore, that Ronald was trying to hold onto his childhood and avoid his responsibilities as an adolescent becomes evident from the fact that it was at this stage that he began to insist that he did not want to attend school, using the excuse that he was having trouble with other children there. There are two hints in the case that support this conclusion. First, the existence of strange marks on his body tended to prevent him from attending school. For instance, when his mother suggested that he should go to school, the message "No" appeared branded on his body while they were discussing the issue. In general, he was not able to communicate his wishes directly to his mother, who resisted his opposition to attending school despite the ordeal that he was undergoing; she simply did not want him to lose the school year that he was already halfway through.

Since Ronald was presumably aware that his mother would not readily let him miss any more school, it is plausible that he may have decided to convince her through means other than directly explaining his wishes to her. Moreover, it is important to note that he was well aware of his mother's spiritualistic beliefs; perhaps through "very special spiritualistic communications, he may have concluded that she might change her mind and obey the message of the spirits." To this end he might have conceived a plan to inflict the marks on himself. Indeed, it is interesting that, several times when the marks seemed to appear spontaneously, he was both near a bathroom where sharp objects are often kept, and also out of the sight of his mother. Thus, he had the opportunity to create "spiritual messages" to convince his superstitious mother. On the other hand, If the marks really appeared or were branded on his body spontaneously, they may have been the result of "a dermatological reaction due to the high level of stress he was undergoing" (Lachman, 1972)—in other words, a somatization of a stressful psychological disorder related to a family conflict that had not been resolved, very much like the somatization of conversion reaction disorders.

There is an additional dimension of the case that ought to be considered in this context. According to the testimony of one witness, Ronald was not doing well at school and was having difficulties with other children. Indeed, some of the paranormal poltergeist-like phenomena began at school, where pieces of furniture reportedly moved around him (interview with Ida Mae by Rueda).[31] Moreover, Ronald's conscious or unconscious intentions to hold onto his childhood and avoid responsibilities at school are evident from the fact that he tried to leave home to go to live with his favorite aunt in Saint Louis—the one who would encourage him to use the Ouija board instead of encouraging him to interact and socialize with other children of his age.

The psychodynamics of the case so far presented lead to the conclusion that the Mount Rainier Exorcism is characterized by many of the psychological dimensions typical of poltergeist cases. That is, we have an adolescent facing a psychological and emotional problem in which he is not in a position to express the conflict openly; therefore, the poltergeist activity may have served the purpose of reinforcing his point of view and providing a release for his stress. In other words, all the elements in the psychological profile of Ronald, the conflictive family and other factors, according to poltergeist researchers, could lead the adolescent to become subject of a poltergeist phenomenon. However, before we address the above poltergeist hypothesis, I will define what a poltergeist is and how it is manifested, in order to facilitate the reader the understanding of this hypothesis as a possible explanatory model for the Mount Rainier Exorcism.

In this regard, Michael Daniels, a famous parapsychologist, provides us with a nice summary of what poltergeists are at his web page, Psychic Science ("About Poltergeists," July 2016):

> *What does "poltergeist" mean?* "Poltergeist" is a German word meaning "noisy spirit." The term is commonly applied to cases in which there are recurrences of spontaneous **physical** phenomena that appear to be paranormal in nature….
>
> *What are poltergeist phenomena?* Typically, poltergeist (RSPK) manifestations involve recurrences of one or more of the following (apparently paranormal) phenomena:
>
> - Opening, closing or banging of doors or windows
> - Movements (including levitation) of domestic objects (e.g., furniture)
> - Sounds of raps or cracking
> - Pinching, scratching or biting of skin
> - Lights or luminous effects
>
> *The "Poltergeist Agent"*: …[P]oltergeist cases appear to be focused around a specific person (occasionally two people). If the family moves home, the phenomena sometimes follow this person (known as the "poltergeist agent") to the new home.
>
> The poltergeist agent is usually a child, teenager, or young adult—most commonly a pre-pubescent or pubescent girl (9–13 years).
>
> In many poltergeist cases, there are complex and emotionally conflicted family dynamics. Often the family has a strict, authoritarian and punitive regime, and may be strongly religious. One widely-accepted theory is that poltergeist phenomena are a psychokinetic manifestation of the agent's intense repressed anger at another, more powerful, family member (who may, directly or indirectly, be the target of the activity). Often, however, the anger seems to be directed at the self, so that the poltergeist agent becomes the victim.

With the above context framed, it is important to note that the Mt. Rainier case shares some of the typical characteristics of family dynamics that are part of conventional cases of poltergeist activity (Gauld and Cornell, 1979).[32]

For instance, in Roll's (1977)[33] collection of cases, the average duration of poltergeist events was within two months; in the Mt. Rainier case, in which the activity began on January 15, 1949, and ended on April 18 of the same year, when the Ritual of Exorcism was said to have freed the boy from the demonic possession, the duration was three months and three days. Another characteristic of the cases collected by Roll is that, although the ages of the agents ranged from 8 to 78, the median age was 13 years. When the ostensible poltergeist phenomena began to appear in the Mt. Rainier case, the boy was 14 years old. The tendency toward adolescent foci is also found in the cases described by Gauld and Cornell.

Another interesting dimension that the Mt. Rainier case had in common with Gauld and Cornell's collection is that the poltergeist outbreaks, in addition to centering on a particular individual known as the focus agent, followed the agent to locations outside the home. In Gauld and Cornell's book, this took place in 42 percent of the cases. Thus, when Ronald was taken to the premises of the Lutheran minister, the latter did not expect the phenomena to be manifested there; however, the poltergeist-like activity did continue to occur, to the surprise of the minister. Also, the phenomena manifested while the boy was at school, as his desk moved around on the schoolroom floor.

In addition, the phenomena followed the adolescent to St. Louis, where the second exorcism took place. Regarding the precipitating events of poltergeist phenomena, William Roll also indicates that, in 38 cases out of 92 with focal persons, the poltergeist events began at a time when there were problems in the family that had to be faced by the focal person. Moreover, in 12 cases the person was ill or subject to unusual psychological stress. Also, as previously noted, in this case Ronald was being subjected to enormous stress as a result of his conflict with his parents regarding school. In addition, as time went on, his favorite aunt, who was not only his aunt but also his playmate, died.

Still another dimension should be considered in the context of Rogo's (1979)[34] assessments of poltergeist cases. Rogo found 8 cases where the poltergeist incidents erupted after a move to a reportedly haunted house or were followed by a mediumistic or spiritualist communication. It is known that Ronald had been involved in some sort of mediumistic communication with his aunt, who taught him how to use the Ouija board in order to communicate with spirits. She had also taught him that, in the absence of a Ouija board, the spirits could try to get through to this world by rapping on the walls (Allen, 1993).[35] Moreover, she told him that the spirits could communicate by entering the consciousness of people around the table. Consequently, as a result of his aunt's teachings, Ronald used to play often with the Ouija board in order to communicate with the spirits. There was family support for this approach, as when the ordeal began, instead of pursuing a medical intervention to cure the boy, the parents instead brought in a spiritualist to perform an ancient ritual.

Furthermore, there are some indications that Ronald may have tried to contact his deceased aunt via the Ouija board after she died. In two poltergeist cases mentioned by Rogo (1979),[36] the incidents began shortly after the death of a close relative or friend. It is important to note that, even though the poltergeist-like phenomena appeared before the death of Ronald's aunt, their frequency increased dramatically after her death.

Irwin (1979)[37] reports that incidences of poltergeist disturbances may initially recur often, but they tend to diminish rapidly after some time. Similarly, in the Mt. Rainier case, the poltergeist-like events diminished as time went by; indeed, most of the dramatic phenomena such as levitation, movement of objects and the like, were reported previous to the second exorcism, which ostensibly freed the boy from his possession. There were, however, some instances of poltergeist activity that seemed to be very stable throughout the entire ordeal and the exorcism, as with the shaking of the mattress in a very dramatic manner that was witnessed by Schulze. Another example is the boy's knowledge of hidden information, an ability of the "possessed" to reveal things of which they could not normally have been aware, as in the identification of hidden religious objects. Also, some of the family members reported that he was able to share information about their private lives. However, reports on the aforementioned phenomena are vague and unclear, appearing as isolated incidents.

John Palmer, a famous parapsychologist, has raised the question in two of his studies about RSPK (recurrent spontaneous psychokinesis), an acronym used by the researcher to designate poltergeist cases. The acronym implies the recurrence of movement of objects by the mind at a distance and the like, such as those manifested in poltergeist cases.

According to Palmer, poltergeist cases might tend to begin with sounds and develop to movements of objects (Palmer, 1974[38]; Pratt & Palmer, 1976[39]). According to his investigation of the cases where we know which came first, 17 began with sounds and 14 with movements. In the Mt. Rainier case, this tendency is also present, as the initial phenomenon began with a dripping noise heard by Ronald and his grandmother in the latter's bedroom. The second sound phenomenon in the case was the shaking of a picture of Christ, as if the wall had been bumped from the back. Other activities in the Mt. Rainier case are consistent with poltergeist-like phenomena.

Similarly, some of the characteristics found in the Mt. Rainier case are associated with ostensible paranormal events such as the movement of objects. In about 90 percent of the cases Roll (1977)[40] mentions, recurrent movement of objects occurs, making it one of the most common features of poltergeist activity. In Gauld and Cornell's (1979)[41] books, 64 percent of cases are marked by the movements of small objects, and 36 percent by the movement of larger objects such as furniture, thus covering the two instances present in the Mt. Rainier case. Initially, however, in this case the movement of objects was mainly related to smaller items such as fruit, as a pear flew the width of Ronald's room; also, a coat on its hanger flew across the room, and a Bible landed at Ronald's feet. Most of the above phenomena, however, were reported by members of the family and not witnessed by anyone else. But then, as the number of incidents increased, larger objects such as a heavy armchair moved, specifically the one in which the Reverend Schulze placed the boy the night he spent at the parsonage.

The occurrence of noises in the form of knocking and scratching sounds was frequent at the initial stages of the exorcism. For instance, that dripping noise, which was heard by Ronald and his grandmother, became a very definite scratching sound under the floorboards near the grandmother's bed by the time Ronald's parents returned home that night. Moreover, when the family suspected that there was, perhaps, a connection between the mysterious sounds and the boy's recently deceased aunt, the mother asked the suspected spirit, "If you are Aunt Dorothy, knock three times," at which point three distinct sounds were heard on the floor. The presence of sounds such as knocking, pounding, rapping, and scratching was found in about half of Gauld and Cornell's collection (1979, p. 387).[42] Furthermore, in 15 percent of the poltergeist cases in that assemblage, there were manifestations of personal assaults such as scratches or bites during the poltergeist activity. In the Mt. Rainier case, there were personal assaults by the supposed entity on the adolescent, through the marks branded on his body in the form of words and letters.

Finally, Roll (1977, p. 405)[43] suggests a psychological mechanism to explain RSPK, based on a survey indicating that, at the time of the poltergeist incidents, the RSPK agent suffered from a poor state of health, either mental or physical. Roll further points out: "The existence of precipitating factors reinforces the impression of pathological conditions which are triggered into overt expression when the situation becomes overtly stressful" (1977, p. 405).[44] Rogo (1979)[45] observes that research conducted by other parapsychologists tends also in this direction, namely, that incidents are related to psychological tension. Among those researchers are Bender (1969),[46] Mischo (1968),[47] and Owen (1969).[48]

As previously indicated, Ronald was undergoing a great deal of stress due to the psychological conflict caused by his refusal to attend school and the corresponding parental pressure on him to change his mind. Also present were the precipitating factors typical in conventional poltergeist cases, such as family changes and the death of his favorite aunt. Moreover, even though he was initially declared to be normal by the psychiatrist who assessed him at the Mental Hygiene Clinic of the University of Maryland, his mental condition worsened after the phenomena began. Indeed, one of the doctors who

;ated him prescribed barbital, which is typically used as an anticonvulsant
ir epileptic seizures or as an inducement to sleep.

So far up to this point, the information presented seems to indicate that
Ronald was very likely the subject of poltergeist activity, which fits some of
the characteristics presented in Gauld and Cornell's and Rogo's case collections. Nevertheless, can these parallels be said to constitute definite proof
that this is a conventional case of poltergeist activity in the context of demonic
possession? In other words, is it necessary to propose a demonic possession
agency in order to explain a conventional poltergeist case?

Regarding such cases, Irwin (1979)[49] has wisely indicated that theories
that have gained wide support from parapsychologists in recent years propose
that poltergeist effects are due to the use of a subconscious PK (subconscious
mind movement of objects at a distance) as a release from considerable psychological tension. Therefore, the demonic possession agency is not needed
to account for the phenomena; we can have recourse to a natural mechanism
which may entirely explain the phenomena surrounding the boy. Is this a
case where the demonic possession hypothesis was introduced later into what
was really just a poltergeist case? Additionally, could demonic possession
cases actually be poltergeist cases masked by religious beliefs?

In this regard, it is helpful to cite the work of Scott Rogo, a parapsychologist who has made a special study of possession phenomena. In his fine
analysis titled *The Poltergeist Experience* (1979),[50] he distinguishes two types of
cases: a conventional poltergeist experience (Type I poltergeist), and a possession
poltergeist experience (Type II poltergeist). There are some features in the Type
II poltergeist event that seem to suggest that some agency is both dependent on
the psyche of the "possessed" and at the same time in some way independent.

In his book, *The Sacred and the Psychic* (1984),[51] Heaney lists these signs
of independence:

1. The ability of the possessed to understand and show fluent skill in
   an unknown or unlearned language (known as xenoglossy).
2. A feeling of horror on the part of the possessed about what is happening to him or her. (In contrast, hysteria cases, it seems, often
   show indifference to the events that center around them.)
3. Transferred possession and simultaneous cure of the possessed; in
   some cases, a possessed person is cured when the possession phenomena take hold of another person, such as a physician or an
   exorcist.
   a. Sudden appearance of paranormal powers in another person
      or in a number of persons, together with
   b. Disappearance of the possession phenomena in the originally possessed person.

4. Some secondary criteria that possibly might have other explanations in situations where the exorcism is successful. In these cases, the possessed spirit is believed to be a deceased human who is seemingly convinced to go on to other tasks while continuing to evolve in the afterlife.

Other signs, according to Heaney, include a horrid stench or a feeling of clammy cold; blasphemy and malicious actions where humans are hurt, harried, or killed; strange matter such as pins being vomited; pernicious happenings frequently when no one else is present, but whose aftereffects can be seen; independent voices coming from a distance while the victim remains unmoving; sensational levitations; violent contortions; and swelling of the body.

Despite all these characteristics that distinguish possession cases from conventional poltergeist events, it is conceivable that the phenomena of a poltergeist nature might be contaminated by the introduction of a causal demonic agent, thus making the person begin to act as if he or she were possessed. Heaney himself acknowledges that, even though parapsychology provides a reasonable theoretical framework to explain demonic possession cases, they can't always be explained entirely via parapsychological mechanisms. As he declares it, "Parapsychology has made it much more difficult in any given case to make dogmatic pronouncements about the reality of possession; however, at the same time, I believe one should hesitate to say also that all possession cases are exclusively cases of pathological hysteria combined with paranormal powers in the possessed" (p. 39).

Scott Rogo (1979)[52] developed a theory that possession cases are examples of the operation of an agency which is part of the victim's own psyche, but which has attained a kind of independence of its own and is thus the cause of the strange phenomena. As he further indicates, "Some split-off portion of the agent's mind" (p. 39) controls the activity of the person's mind. He uses as evidence experiences like those of Alexandra David-Neel in Tibet, who tried to invoke the apparition of a monk and was amazed when the figure did appear. It took six months of struggle to rid herself of this phantom creature, which was also seen by one other person. Likewise, Rogo uses data from out-of-body experience (OBE) studies in which part of the person's personality separates as if into a kind of ex-somatic state. According to this theory, possession phenomena are caused by a quasi-independent agency that is ultimately traceable to the person's own psyche, in the form of its dark side.

Even though Rogo admits that the set of manifestations of a PK (psychokinesis, the paranormal influence of the mind on physical events and processes) phenomenon differentiates poltergeist cases from possession pol-

st cases, he also points out that some possession poltergeist events may
: from suggestion, caused by what he then calls the "delusion of posses-
' which arises later in a poltergeist case. For instance, he makes reference
ie Mt. Rainier case, in which the onset of possession was preceded by six
:ks by the PK effects. He also points out, "It was only after the family
;an to think in terms of demonic possession that the boy began to manifest
e classical symptoms; this certainly looks as though suggestion was the
,ot of the possession syndrome" (p. 22). In other words, if we call the devil,
/e will see him, but in the form of the manifestations of the victim's ideas of
1im—that is, the boy began acting as a possessed person is "supposed" to
act. It is likely that the family's superstitious beliefs about what was taking
place with Ronald may have triggered the possession case. Maybe what began
with obsession and poltergeist phenomena was transformed into possession
by the decision to exorcise. If there had been no exorcism, perhaps the Mt.
Rainier case would never have happened in the way that it did.

In support of the above assertion that the introduction of exorcism into
the case may have triggered possession, there are indications in the Jesuit
Report that, up to March 15, before the exorcism began, the phenomena
reported had been obsession, that is, exterior to the boy (J.R., p. 8).

Secondly, by reading the Jesuit Report, as soon as the exorcism began
on March 16, obsession changed to possession, and classical signs of demonic
possession began to manifest (J.R., p. 16). This is another important dimension, suggesting that the adolescent may have been motivated to remain possessed. For instance, the Jesuit Report indicates that Easter Monday, April 18,
was the worst day and the exorcists were becoming thoroughly discouraged.
As the Jesuit Report relates: "There was no response to the 'Praecipio' except
taunting remarks to the exorcists. Everyone, including R, was becoming weary
of the long performance. R did not begin to sleep until midnight. The Fathers
left the Hospital at 12:45 p.m." (J.R., p. 26).

It is interesting to see that, when they reached that point of exhaustion,
the boy may have noticed and decided to put an end to the ordeal of possession, one that he may have created in his mind, along with the participation
of those who had paid him too much attention. This was, indeed, the day
when he was liberated from the possession by the exorcists. This timeline
readily leads one to express some reservations about the authenticity of this
case.

Along these same lines, Oesterreich (1966) has indicated that the general
view of possession current at the time or in the patient's circle "immediately
causes these compulsions to be interpreted as a second individuality. According to the disposition of the person affected, this may easily and automatically
lead to imaginative identification with the second personality; the autosug-
gestion resulting from distress of mind must favor this.... [M]uch more prob-

able is that it was often rather the conviction of being possessed which brought about a real division of the mind" (p. 91).

Oesterreich (1966)[53] further declares: "The reign of superstition was responsible for the fact, as the abundance of documents at our disposal show at every step that the mildest compulsions were immediately taken for demoniacal" (p. 91). It is important to note that the belief in possession is not as common as it used to be in the past, although there are still social and religious circles where the belief in possession or spirit possession is very much engraved and perhaps reflected in a more pronounced manner, including in fundamentalist religious groups such as the Pentecostals.

The Mt. Rainier case constitutes a good example of how superstition and belief in demonic possession may combine to create a real case of demonic possession. In this regard, Oesterreich (1966)[54] observes, "At so primitive levels of culture and with patients of such enhanced autosuggestibility, it is not surprising that a state of possession should readily arise" (p. 95).

Another dimension that is worth considering relates to Rogo's comment that poltergeist and possession poltergeist events also show different psychological dimensions, although he does not clearly delineate these differences. Nevertheless, it is plausible that their psychological atmospheres differ significantly in terms of the religious elements introduced in the possession poltergeist event, which may lead a conventional poltergeist case to become an actual case of demonic possession. Once the religious element of demonic possession is embedded in the case, the psychological atmosphere changes and the level of autosuggestibility increases, thus triggering demonic possession onto the adolescent. It is important to note in support of this assertion that, when the Mt. Rainier case was in the hands of the Lutheran minister, who was not very sympathetic to the demonic agency hypothesis, neither the family nor anyone else involved made the slightest mention of possession or the devil. It was only later, when the Catholic ministers got involved, that the possession case began. It was they who began to search for signs of possession, as indicated in the Roman Ritual. The poltergeist hypothesis embraced by the Lutheran minister was left to the side, to be replaced by the new hypothesis proposed by the Catholic priest who decided to conduct an exorcism.

Once the idea of demonic possession was proposed to the family by the priest, who had initially believed that the phenomena had been caused by Ronald's recently deceased aunt, their commitment to that idea was triggered and demonic possession began. The mind of the adolescent began to manifest the new signs that fit the ideas about demonic possession. This brings to mind the case of an adolescent female member of a Pentecostal church where I used to attend services, who at one point behaved aggressively towards a classmate in Sunday school; she began to act as possessed when some members of the church told her that her act had been caused by the devil, who had entered her mind. Suggestion is a powerful tool in inducing beliefs and somatizations. For instance, high levels of suggestibility may lead people to believe odd things, such as when women who are not pregnant, but believe that they are, manifest symptoms of pregnancy such as a swollen belly, enlarged breasts, and even the sensation of fetal movement. The technical name for this condition is known pseudocyesis (false pregnancy); in this condition, psychological factors may trick the body of a woman into "thinking" that she is pregnant.

The telekinetic force of poltergeist cases may be redirected toward religious rituals or objects. As noted by Thurston (1953),[55] just as the demoniacs are violently antireligious, a well-known propensity of the poltergeist is to destroy or telekinetically affect religious objects.

To sum up, the introduction of the religious element into a conventional poltergeist case brings into play a new psychological dimension, which, in turn, makes this a case of possession poltergeist. Consequently, it may be said that Type I and II poltergeist cases are basically the same, except that the religious element in the second type brings into play new telekinetic forces.

So far, the Mt. Rainier case has been evaluated in the context of the poltergeist hypothesis, as that is where it appears to fit best. However, it becomes a Type II poltergeist case once the religious element of demonic agency is introduced later on. There are, indeed, some dimensions of the case, such as the testimony of the Reverend Schulze, that seem to indicate that it may have been a genuine poltergeist case and not simply the result of fraud. Some phenomena, which appear to be very suggestive of paranormal activity, cannot be entirely explained by fraud or a psychological disturbance.

At the same time, some may argue that, despite his skepticism, the Reverend Schulze was a believer in the paranormal, since he had followed the work of J.B. Rhine at Duke; thus he may have led himself to believe that he was witnessing a genuine paranormal phenomenon. Yet the way he managed the case does not indicate that he was an easy person to fool or particularly susceptible to the phenomena he witnessed; it would have been difficult to deceive a person with his scientific attitude. Up to the time when I interviewed him, he remained skeptical regarding the existence of a preternatural agency in this case, although he continued to believe that he had witnessed phenomena that he could not explain scientifically. When he was asked about his belief in parapsychology, he replied, "I was not a believer in parapsychology, even though I had followed with most interest the work of J.B. Rhine at Duke, and I do think I witnessed genuine phenomena that I could not account for.... I even at some time on the case considered the criteria used by Catholics to diagnose cases of demonic possession; however, I never saw any of those signs on this particular case" (interview with the Reverend Schulze, 1990). I would conclude that all elements seem to be strongly suggestive that some type of poltergeist activity, as theorized by experts on parapsychology, may have taken place. However, still in spite of the strong similarities between poltergeist cases and the Mount Rainier Exorcism, the poltergeist hypothesis would stand, if all the phenomena actually took place and the ostensible phenomena reported on the cases is truthful. This would in turn serve the parapsychological claims that paranormal phenomena actually exist. However, skeptical researchers would believe this case does not fit the current laws of the limiting principles of science, and another causal hypothesis may be held accountable in this case.

14

The Devil in Disguise
The Diabolical Possession Agency Hypothesis

Can demons possess humans? Interestingly, many people believe even today that evil spirits, called demons, can take over people's bodies. This idea, which was widely accepted in Europe hundreds of years ago, is still believed by many in areas of Africa where the influence of Christianity is not strong. It is also a growing belief in America. A study revealed that about one-third of all Americans believe that demons can take over the bodies of people. What does that mean in terms of teachings of the Bible?

The Bible clearly indicates that evil spirits exist (James 2:19). They are called "devils" in the King James Version, and "demons" in other translations. These devils, or demons, must not be confused with the Devil, Satan, or the Tempter (Matthew 4:11). There is only one Devil, but there are many demons. Thus, in the Bible, we learn that demons entered into people and controlled them (Matthew 8:28–34). Being under the power of Satan (Beelzebub), the chief of all evil spirits (Matthew 12:24), they often caused sickness in the people they entered, such as an inability to speak or see (Matthew 12:22); insanity or madness (Luke 8:26–36); personal injuries (Mark 9:14–26); and other bodily infirmities (Luke 13:11–17).

These demons also knew who Jesus was. They knew why He had come into the world: eternal punishment (Matthew 8:29). This clearly shows that demons are not diseases, as some have suggested. They are spirit beings who think, speak, and act. Jesus often cast demons out of people (Matthew 8:16). He also gave the ability to cast out demons to His apostles (Luke 10:17; Mark 16:17–18; Acts 5:16; 8:7; 16:16; 19:12). The apostles were able to give miraculous gifts to others by laying their hands on them (Acts 6:6–8; 8:14–21; 19:1:6) this included the power to cast out demons (Acts 8:5–8).

An account of Jesus' casting out a demon is found in Mark 5:1–20. When Jesus came to the country of the Gadarenes, he was met by a man who had an "unclean spirit" (that is, a demon). This demon-possessed man lived in the tombs. He wore no clothes. He was not in his right mind. He cried day and night and cut himself with stones. He also had great strength. When others bound him with chains, he broke them and escaped. The evil spirit in the man knew who Jesus was and begged Him not to torment him. Jesus asked the evil spirit, "What is thy name?" He replied, "My name is Legion; for we are many." When Jesus commanded the demons to come out of the man, they begged him to send them into pigs that were feeding nearby. Jesus did so, the pigs ran to the cliff, fell into the sea, and drowned. When the people of the area came to Jesus, they saw this man "sitting, clothed, and in his right mind." When the demon was cast out, the man was restored to health of body and mind. In short, the Bible teaches us that demons exist and that, as a sign of their power and rebellion against God, they possess human beings in order to influence and control them so that their minds become evil.

However, before initiating an evaluation, based on the hypothesis of diabolic agency, of the Mount Rainier case, on which the film *The Exorcist* was based, it is important to note and understand that "demonic possession" is a dogma or belief of the Catholic Church that has been embraced up to the present time; moreover, as we have previously indicated, it was a widely accepted belief in the time of Jesus, who actually performed at least one exorcism. Since we have to believe in the existence of the demon as a real entity in order to believe that demonic possession can actually occur at the present time, my analysis of the case from this perspective will be done in the context of this dogma. Since the existence of demons can neither be proven nor disproven in an indisputable manner, at this point we will depend on faith in analyzing this case, if we want to allow for a possible diagnosis of demonic possession intended to harm human beings and make them rebel against God. The existence of demons comes to us, after all, as a result of biblical teachings.

Regarding the existence of demonic possession and the reality of exorcism, John Warwick Montgomery declared: "The reality of exorcism thus depends squarely on the reality of [demons] or demon possession. If there is no personal supernatural evil, then clearly there are no demons to possess people, no genuine exorcisms of demons. Moreover, even if demons exist, if they did not enter and control human personalities, exorcism would be purposeless. The exorcist claims to be a physician for souls—not a general practitioner but a specialist—and the validity of his activity depends on whether the particular disease he aims to cure really exists" (p. 5).[1]

In order to determine if the Mount Rainier incident is a genuine case of demonic possession, or at least meets the standards for such as established by the Catholic Church, I will now present some historical and theological information in order to frame the Mount Rainier case in terms of Catholic Church dogma and its diagnostic tool, the Roman Ritual. While we have already seen that the Bible indisputably accepts the existence of demons and their ability to possess humans, how would such a diagnosis come about? Theologians from the Catholic Church developed the Roman Ritual in 1914 for this purpose, and a revised version was presented in 1999.

The first question is why, if the Devil exists, would he would be interested in possessing human beings? Let us look at some of the history or the origin of this creature. According to theologians such as Father Gabriele Amorth, Chief Exorcist of Rome:

> Satan was the most perfect being created by the hands of God. His God-given authority and superiority over the other angels are recognized by all, so he thought that he had the same authority over everything that God was creating. Satan tried to understand all of creation but could not, because all the plan of creation was oriented toward Christ. Until Christ came into the world, God's plan could not be revealed in its entirety. Hence Satan's rebellion. He wanted to continue to be the absolute first, the center of creation, even if it meant opposing God's design. This is why Satan continually tries to dominate the world ("the whole world is in the power of the evil one," I John 5:19). Beginning with our forefathers, he seeks to enslave men by making them obey him and disobey God. He was successful with our forefathers, Adam and Eve, and he hoped to continue with all men with the help of "a third of the angels," who, according to the book of Revelation, followed him in rebellion against God (p. 2).[2]

As a result of the Devil's rebellion against God, Revelation tells us that demons were hurled down to earth. Here, then, the Devil, who decided to continue with his rebellion, tried to make man part of it. This would be achieved by inducing humans to disobey God, or influencing or possessing them to do so.

In sum, we know that Satan and demons do exist, according to the Bible and Church dogma. Similarly, we know that they are disembodied spirits working in the spiritual realm who desire to, and are able to, dwell in humans (and also animals) to influence their bodies and minds for evil; while they vary in power and authority, they are all more powerful than man, and can be controlled or cast out only by the authority of the Lord Jesus Christ. But how much power does a devil have over a Christian? Can devils or demons control a believer as they can a "lost person"?

The Bible mentions two basic types of Satanic or demonic influence or control over men:

1. Satanic or Demonic Oppression, where Satan or devils contact and influence people externally—from the outside in.
2. Demon Indwelling or Possession, where the devils actually dwell inside the person, influencing and manipulating him or her internally—from the inside out.

In the case of Demonic Possession in this book, I will be dealing with the second type of demonic influence.

At the same time, the demon uses several different strategies to influence, control, or possess humans. These different categories are presented by Father Amorth[3] thus:

Temptation: Ordinary activity. "Temptation," the most common activity of the demons, is directed against all men.

External physical pain caused by Satan: We know of this from many lives of the saints. We know that Saint Paul of the Cross, the Curé of Ars, Padre Pio, and many others were beaten, flogged, and pummeled by demons.

Diabolic oppression: Symptoms vary from a very serious to a mild illness. There is no possession, loss of consciousness, or involuntary action or word. The Bible gives us many examples of oppression, one of them being Job. He was not possessed, but he lost his children, his goods, and his health.

Diabolic obsession: Symptoms include sudden attacks, at times ongoing, of obsessive thoughts, sometimes rationally absurd but of such nature that the victim is unable to free himself. Therefore, the obsessed person lives in a perpetual state of prostration or desperation, and may attempt suicide. Almost always obsession influences dreams.

Demonic possession: This occurs when Satan takes full possession of the body (not the soul); he speaks and acts without the knowledge or consent of the victim, who, therefore, is morally blameless. It is the gravest and most spectacular form of demonic affliction.

Possession by Stages

Now, what are the steps in the particular case of demonic possession? My studies with several experts on the topic are summarized as follows:

Manifestation

In this stage, a person will unintentionally invite the demonic force in. There are said to be many different ways for this to happen, the most common being playing with the Ouija board, performing séances, and consulting Tarot cards. The demon will be attracted to individuals who are weak-minded or exhibit low self-esteem. People who are alcoholics, drug addicts, or sex addicts may be easy targets as well.

Note: In the Mount Rainier exorcism, Ronald used the Ouija board to contact his deceased aunt.

Infestation

At this level, the demon will start using what may seem like typical intelligent haunting signs. The demon may present itself as the ghost of a loved one or even an angel. The point is to gain trust, so that the demon may influence the person and finally take full control. Some signs of demonic infestation include rappings, shadows, shadow-like figures that move with no explanation, the sounds of footsteps, or weird liquids that seep through the floor or walls.

Note: In the Mount Rainier case, the demons appeared to answer questions of the deceased aunt by knocking on wood and received responses with similar sounds.

Oppression

When an individual is under demonic oppression, the demon starts to affect the person psychologically, psychically, and emotionally. The purpose is to cause the individual to give up the fight or will to live and damn his or her soul; this may be accomplished by suicide.

Note: Emotionally, Ronald underwent episodes of extreme anger and became very aggressive toward those around him.

Possession

When an individual hits this level, it is called full possession. The demon or devil now has control over the person's thoughts, emotions, and behavior. The evil spirit is frequently, if not constantly, in charge. If or when the individuals are in control of their own bodies, they may hear evil voices either threatening them or telling them what to do at all time. Apparently, according to many witnesses and the priest who performed the exorcism, Ronald was possessed by the Devil once the exorcism began.

In the particular case of the Mount Rainier Exorcism, Ronald seems to have suffered from all of the above stages. However, we will now consider two of them. First was the Infestation stage that was evaluated by Father William Bowdern as being part of the issue. He knew from family reports that phenomena such as the sound of footsteps and weird liquids seeping through the floor or walls had been observed. Second was the Obsession stage, which reflects the terrible emotional turmoil that Ronald was experiencing. Although this is a stage that can also be explained by psychological or psychiatric mechanisms, experts on demonic possession attribute it to the influence of the demon who is intending to move into possession of the victim.

It was at this point that Father Bowdern made the decision to carry out an exorcism as a preventive or prophylactic measure. However, the more cautious Archbishop was reluctant to approve it. What if it turned out to be a terrible mistake to proceed with an exorcism, in the absence of the actual signs of possession, as called for by the Roman Ritual? Bowdern defended his decision to exorcise the adolescent, as he was absolutely convinced that this was an actual case of demonic possession.

Regarding the Mount Rainier case, Father Bowdern, the real exorcist, wrote to William Peter Blatty: "I can assure you of one thing; the case in which I was involved was the real thing [possession]. I had no doubt about it then and I have no doubt about it now" (Brian, 1982, p. 183).[4]

Moreover, Father John Nicola,[5] who was a consultant for the film *The Exorcist*, supported the diabolical agency hypothesis held by Bowdern. In his book *Diabolical Possession and Exorcism* (1974), he noted that there were abundant written accounts and innumerable witnesses, nearly all of whom, as a result of their experiences in the case, believed that the devil had indeed possessed the young adolescent. It is important to note that Father Nicola had access to firsthand information from witnesses, as well as to accounts and taped reports of hospital staff and Ronald's family members, all of whom witnessed some of the phenomena. All this evidence led Father Nicola to the conclusion that this was a genuine case of demonic possession. Therefore, according to him, the case showed the signs of possession in a conclusive manner, to the point where all alternative explanations of causality could be discarded.

Also, according to Allen (1993), author of the book *Possessed*,[6] Father Nicola actually believed that Ronald was diabolically possessed. As for Father Bowdern, he seems to have come to the same conclusion soon after he began to perform the exorcism. According to the diary kept by one of the priests during the exorcism, "up to this time everything had been obsession but as soon as the exorcism began March 16, possession began" (Cortes, 1975, p. 75).[7] Previous to the exorcism, the phenomena surrounding the boy initially resembled the classical progression from infestation to obsession or invasion of the individual, as happens in diabolical possession. During this stage, the Devil attacks the individual in a manner that is both intense and invisible, such that there can be no doubt of his presence and activity (Balducci, 1990, p. 110).[8] For instance, the brandings and marks that later appeared on the boy's body resembled the affliction that sometimes takes place in cases of obsession. For Bowdern the progression from infestation to obsession was an indication that the boy was near the next step, which is possession. In order to prevent that from happening, he decided to go ahead and request the Archbishop for permission to perform an exorcism. Allen quotes Bowdern as having said, "Maybe we can stop it here" (p. 70).

Furthermore, he adds: "Fathers Bishop and Bowdern decided to ask the local Archbishop Ritter to find and appoint an exorcist to perform the exorcism before a demon would enter Robbie" (p. 70). As the J.R. relates: "Permission was granted by the Most Reverend Archbishop Joseph E. Ritter that

Father William S. Bowdern, S.J., Pastor of the College Church in St. Louis might read the prayers of exorcism according to the Roman Ritual" (J.R., p. 7).

Evidently, Bowdern had gathered insufficient evidence to diagnose the case as demonic possession; however, he proceeded to ask the Archbishop for permission to perform an exorcism on Ronald. The evidence led Father Bowdern to conclude that he was dealing with a case of obsession, but still he decided to proceed with an exorcism. It is important to note that his conclusion came after having examined this case in the light of the Roman Ritual's rules and observations. In this regard, the Roman Ritual[9] warns that "an exorcist should not believe too readily that a person is possessed by an evil spirit for the person might be suffering from mental illness." Along these lines, according to the Vatican guidelines, issued in 1999, "the person who claims to be possessed must be evaluated by doctors to rule out a mental or physical illness."[10] Moreover, with our current more advanced knowledge of psychological and psychiatric pathology, many times a person just needs spiritual or medical help, especially if drugs or other addictions are present. Currently, the Catholic Church generally advises that after the need of the person has been determined then the appropriate help will be met. In the circumstance of spiritual help, prayers may be offered, or the laying on of hands or a counseling session may be prescribed.

Furthermore, Father Bowdern, who asked for the permission to perform the exorcism, followed the very vague criteria stated in the Roman Ritual to determine his diagnosis of obsession, which in his opinion, based on no experience in cases of demonic possession and exorcism, would turn into a case of possession. What are the criteria that he used to proceed with the exorcism? Evidence in this regard will be evaluated, in the next sections, as to what he had at hand as evidence to support his decision for an exorcism to be performed on Ronald.

The Granting of Permission to Provide the Wrong Medicine for the Wrong Illness

Archbishop Ritter, to whom Bowdern had asked for permission to perform the exorcism, had not observed the phenomena nor the symptoms surrounding the adolescent. Evidently, the archbishop was aware that the case did not meet the standards established by the Roman Ritual for cases of demonic possession, except what had been reported to him verbally by Father William Bowdern. Moreover, no medical, psychological or psychiatric evaluation had been presented to him, as the guidelines of the Vatican require for cases of demonic possession. Nevertheless, although the boy did not exhibit the conventional signs indicative of possession mentioned in the Ritual, Archbishop Ritter still granted the permission to Father Bowdern to proceed with an exorcism.

A Case of Religious Medicine with a Wrong Diagnosis

It is important to note that in the previous exorcism, performed on Ronald by Father Hughes, the 14-year-old adolescent showed none of the traditional signs of diabolical possession cited in the Roman Ritual. Thus we have a second wrong religious diagnosis for a spiritual illness. In other words, they asked for the wrong treatment for the wrong condition, "an exorcism for a case of obsession in both cases." In both the first and second exorcisms, we have a violation of the essential rules and recommendations of the Roman Ritual and the guidelines of the Vatican for cases of demonic possession.

However, in order to support his case and perform the exorcism, Father Bowdern consulted books and theological works on demonic possession to find an answer. His readings of the theological works "strengthened him in thinking," that he should proceed with the exorcism, says Thomas Allen, in his book *Possessed* (p. 71); his study of the case showed the classical progression from infestation to obsession. Therefore, the next step of the progression would indeed be "possession," according to the theological works he had read. With his information in hand, Bowdern decided to request the performance of an exorcism on Ronald in order to stop the apparent progression from obsession to possession—in other words, to prevent actual possession from happening. The archbishop did grant permission to proceed, appointing Father Bowdern as the exorcist in the case, even while knowing that, at that stage, it was an issue of obsession, not of possession. In this regard, Allen declared: "He had no conclusive way to prove that Robbie was possessed or in an imminent danger of being possessed. The boy showed none of the traditional signs cited in the Roman Ritual" (p. 81).

In sum, as previously mentioned, the boy was not diabolically possessed, at least in terms of the standards of the Roman Ritual, at the time when Bowdern requested that an exorcism be performed on him. The diagnosis was, according to Bowdern himself, "obsession." In order to prevent possession (the next step) from taking place, the archbishop authorized the exorcism, being aware that the boy was in danger of presenting the traditional signs of possession cited in the Ritual, or in imminent danger of being possessed. In other words, it was a prophylactic or preventive measure. At the same time, the priest who requested the exorcism did break the rules of the Roman Ritual.

If the archbishop was aware that Ronald did not actually show the signs indicative of possession mentioned in the Ritual, nor was he in imminent danger of being possessed, why, then, did he authorize the exorcism? He was aware, according to Allen, that "if the boy was suffering from mental illness rather than diabolical possession, an exorcism would do no good and could even worsen his condition" (p. 81). There is no answer to this question, according to Allen, who simply notes the dilemma faced by the archbishop as to "whether or not to authorize the exorcism" (p. 79). Perhaps the decision to authorize the exorcism was made under the assumption that Ronald was probably possessed, or perhaps the archbishop accepted Father Bowdern's supposition that Ronald suffered from obsession and would probably reach the next level of possession in the absence of an exorcism. At any rate, by Allen's account, it is not clear what really led the archbishop to grant permission to perform an exorcism on Ronald in spite of its contraindications.

The information that possession actually began at the same time as the exorcism indicates that there was a change in the situation and in the diagnosis: The progression from obsession to possession, which Bowdern was trying to prevent with the exorcism, did take place. According to witnesses, instead of just attacking Ronald with the marks on his body, the devil took the next step of invading Ronald's body at the very moment the treatment that was supposed to end the ordeal began. The traditional progression from infestation through obsession to possession took place, even as the third level of extraordinary diabolical possession (Balducci, 1985) occurred.

Now, the devil was within Ronald's body, over which he had taken control. The progression from obsession to possession must have been marked by changes in the personality and phenomena surrounding the 14-year-old boy. Exactly what were the changes in the symptoms and phenomena that led Father Bowdern to reach this conclusion? What were the parameters used by the Roman Ritual and Father Bowdern to diagnose the case as possession, once the priest had started the exorcism? Originally, when Father Bowdern was introduced to the case and evaluated it, he personally had not witnessed any of the phenomena or supernatural activity reportedly surrounding the adolescent. Moreover, as has been previously noted, Ronald did not exhibit any of the conventional signs indicative of possession mentioned in the Ritual, which Father Bowdern had consulted for guidance. Finally, there was a lack of evidence for the diagnosis of demonic possession. So what did he have at hand to move from the idea of demonic obsession to that of possession? Not much, but previous to the exorcism, he was relying simply on the family accounts as they had related them to him. When Father Bowdern asked his assistant, Father Bishop, to evaluate the case with him, they had to wonder, "What do we have here?" Their response was, "Maybe not enough" (Allen, 1993, p. 69).

The evidence that Father Bowdern and his assistant had gathered so far was too weak to make a case for demonic possession. The very little proof they had handy, indicative of demonic influence, was the apparent rejection of religious objects by the adolescent boy. For instance, religious objects that had been pinned down near the boy had been found disturbed and thrown on the floor; this sort of activity is considered by some theologians as a sign of demonic influence (Balducci, 1990). Moreover, there was the report of Father Bishop, who had witnessed a poltergeist-like phenomenon when he saw Ronald moving dramatically back and forth in the bed, along with additional family reports chronicling similar phenomena that had taken place in Maryland.

Based on the information he had at hand, Father William Bowdern attempted to make a diagnosis of demonic obsession instead, which in his opinion would lead, sooner or later, to demonic possession. He knew that, by the standards of the Roman Ritual, he did not have sufficient evidence to make a case for possession. But if it was not possession, then what kind of demonic influence did the symptoms represent? His inference of obsession demonstrated his lack of experience in cases of possession. Having taken what could be called a crash course on demonic possession, he based his conclusion that an exorcism would end the problem on relatively weak evidence, such as the family account of poltergeist-like events that took place in Maryland, as recorded by Father Bishop in his diary. These phenomena provided the elements for the diagnosis, along with the mark appearing later on the boy's body that seemed to be an attack by the devil.

Moreover, it is important to repeat that Father Bowdern based his diagnosis of the case almost entirely on the family's account of the events that took place in Maryland, even though he and his assistant had not witnessed any of them. Thus, as Cortes has indicated (1975), they appeared to be very credulous in accepting as true events that they had never witnessed, and rendering a diagnosis based on them. More surprisingly, the archbishop then authorized an exorcism based on family reports of symptoms that the priests themselves had never witnessed. Many of the strange phenomena that took place, such as the movement of objects and the signs of marks on the adolescent's body, were mostly reported by Ronald to his parents and the priests, but Father Bowdern never actually witnessed them. For instance, when Father Bowdern was initially brought to the house to see Ronald, a religious object or reliquary and a bottle of holy water that the priests had previously placed in Ronald's room were disturbed. In both cases, however, the priests did not witness the events. When they were pinned down in the room, in full view of the priests, nothing happened. As the Jesuit Report indicates:

> Father Bowdern read the Novena prayer of St. Francis Xavier and then blessed R. with the relic (a piece of bone from the forearm of St. Francis Xavier). Then *** crucifix reliquary was safety-pinned under R's pillow. There was no shaking of the mat-

tress or scratching at this time. After the above blessing the group if observers went downstairs to review some of the history of the case, when a loud crash was heard in R's bedroom. The boy was dozing when the bottle of St. Ignatius holy water was thrown from a table two feet from R's room. A bookcase was moved from alongside the bed and turned completely around facing the entrance to the room. The stool at the dressing table moved from the table to the bed, about two feet. The stool was moved back to its position and in a few moments, it was turned over. Mother and R. were in bed when crucifix with relics was moved from under the pillow to the foot of the bed. The relic of St. Margaret Mary was lost in the room (J.R., pp. 5–6).

It is important to note that, shortly before the reliquary was placed under Ronald's pillow, the relic of St. Margaret Mary that was under the pillow of his bed had levitated, according to the boy; the safety pin had come unfastened, and the relic had risen from the pillow, sailed across the room and struck a mirror. The event had taken place while he was in his bedroom by himself and his parents and the priests were downstairs, out of view of where the phenomena took place.

To sum up this event: After the reliquary was pinned down under Robbie's pillow by Father Bowdern, nothing more happened, and the priests were about to leave the house. From upstairs came a loud sound, leading everybody to rush again to the boy's room. He said that a beaker of holy water, left there by Father Bishop, had flown from a table and landed several feet away.

Again, the phenomenon reported by the boy took place out of the view of the family and the priests, happening only after they had left his room. This type of account represented a frequent pattern of events, including a lot of the phenomena reported by Bishop in his diary and used for background information on the case. Neither the family nor the priests ever witnessed most of the phenomena reported by the boy. Nevertheless, the information provided by the 14-year-old was taken by the diarist as true happenings, accepted with an unquestioning mind. Throughout Allen's account of the case history and the Jesuit Report, the pattern in common was that a strange event would happen to the boy while he was by himself somewhere in the house or his room; he would yell, and somebody would rush up to his room and assist him; but none of these who assisted him witnessed any of the phenomena reported to them by the boy.

To recapitulate, when Father Bowdern initially evaluated the Mount Rainier case based on the Roman Ritual, he found that he did not have sufficient evidence to render a possession diagnosis, since the boy did not manifest conventional signs of possession as cited in the Ritual. Lacking sufficient evidence for a case of demonic possession of Ronald, he went on to study further both the Roman Ritual and historical cases. Then he began to search for answers to explain the phenomenology of the case by consulting theological works to enlighten him. Unfortunately, his assessment depended mostly on the accounts of the case as they were related to him by the family. The family, however, was not a reliable source of information, since they were very superstitious, even going to the point of organizing spiritualistic séances in order to heal the adolescent from his possession. It is important to note that a lot of the phenomena that allegedly took place around the 14-year-old, reported to the diarist by the family, contained information family members had not actually witnessed themselves; rather, they relied on the boy's reports. Yet the information as provided by the family was taken as valid in the determination of the situation as a case of obsession, later turning into a case of demonic possession.

As I have previously indicated, the only evidence Father Bowdern had at hand when he initiated his diagnosis of the case was the apparent aversion of the boy to religious relics; for instance, when he found that a relic placed on the boy's bed had been disturbed, he used this sign as evidence of his diagnosis, even though he had not witnessed the event himself. Moreover, he used the account by his assistant, Father Bishop—who had reported witnessing phenomena such as the shaking of the mattress and the appearance of scratches on the boy's abdomen—although he had not actually seen these marks as they were being made, but only after they appeared and had been reported to him.

The point that I want to make, regarding the procedure used to diagnose the case as one of demonic obsession-possession, is that the priests' investigation was poorly conducted and lacked the precautions called for in this type of case by the Roman Ritual. Furthermore, Father Bowdern appeared credulous to the point of gullibility regarding the events reported to him by the family and his assistant. Neither Thomas Allen's account nor the Jesuit Report tell us whether the priests even sought out alternative hypotheses to explain the case; instead, it seems that they went straight for the supernatural explanation, despite the weak evidence at hand. Moreover, as when the Reverend Schulze worked on the case, nobody ever consulted a medical authority in order to rule out a psychological or medical condition that might have explained the reported phenomena. The priest and his assistant just proceeded with some brief research into the case based on secondhand reports from the family and the diarist. As Allen observes, "In their hasty research between Saturday, March 12, and Tuesday, March 15, they learned enough about exorcism to decide that neither of them was the priest for the task" (p. 71).

According to the chronology of events, Father Bowdern heard about the case on March 10 from Father Bishop, a close friend. The next day, Friday, March 11, Bishop invited Bowdern to visit the boy with him. They did so around 10 p.m. that same day. Once they arrived at the house, Father Bowdern chatted briefly with Ronald, who went off to sleep soon after that, around 11:00 p.m.

Shortly thereafter, a strange phenomenon allegedly took place, while the boy was by himself in his room: a relic rose from the pillow, sailed across the room, and struck a mirror, whereupon Ronald yelled for help and Bowdern and Bishop dashed upstairs to assist him. However, they did not witness the phenomenon themselves.

Moreover, when they were about to leave the house, a loud noise came from the stairs, and again everyone converged on the boy's room. He reported that a bottle of holy water, which had been left in the room, flew from a table and landed six feet away. It is important to note that both of these events, which took place during a period of an hour and a half, happened during Bowdern's first visit to the house, but neither of them was witnessed directly by either the priest or his assistant. This was the same day that Father Bishop started to collect background information on the "Case Study," as he called it in his diary, the Jesuit Report, which contained mostly the family's account of events prior to the involvement of the priests. It was mostly a chronological account of the events that had started back in January of 1949.

Another interesting aspect of this first visit by the priest to the family is the way Father Bowdern dealt with these initial phenomena that he had not personally witnessed. For instance, soon after the bottle of holy water reportedly levitated, the priest held a rosary under the boy's neck and recited the rosary, starting with the words "Deliver us from evil," which, according to Thomas Allen, is a mild form of exorcism. In other words, even in the total absence of evidence to render a diagnosis of demonic possession, the priest proceeded with a mild exorcism, through which he may well have triggered the idea of demonic possession in the boy's mind; in turn, he may have started to act as if he were possessed. This also suggests that at this stage, without having consulted the guidelines of the Roman Ritual to determine if demonic possession was involved, Father Bowdern already believed that there was something diabolical about the case, perhaps even to the extent of possession. This is a crucial moment, where the idea of possession is introduced. In response to the possibility of possession, the family organized a spiritualist séance to discourage the spirit of the recently deceased aunt from interfering in the boy's life, according to their belief that she was the one responsible for the phenomena surrounding the boy.

According to the chronology of events, Allen indicates that, between March 12 and 15, both the priest and his assistant had learned enough about the concept of demonic possession to persuade them that they did not want to be the boy's exorcist. This is clearly an indication of their acknowledgment that they lacked experience in this type of case, as well as their decision, made in just three days, that this was indeed a case of demonic possession that called for an exorcism. However, there is no indication at this point that they had followed the guidelines of the Ritual indicating that psychological or medical causes ought to be ruled out before proceeding to an exorcism. Although at one point the adolescent was placed at the Alexian Brothers Hospital in St. Louis, Missouri, it is not clear as to whether or not a medical evaluation of Ronald was even conducted or that they consulted a medical authority, a procedure that had been followed carefully by the Lutheran minister who had dealt with the case earlier. In other words, they took a "crash course" on demonic possession in four days, thereby becoming "experts" capable of diagnosing the case as one of demonic possession requiring an exorcism.

Also, in just a few days, without a medical report on hand, they obtained permission from the archbishop to proceed with an exorcism. It took them only a weekend plus two business days to start the ritual. Interestingly, what had been a case of obsession turned into possession as soon as the exorcism began. The Canon Law and the Roman Ritual indicate that possession ought to be diagnosed and medical conditions ruled out before proceeding with exorcism. Solemn exorcisms, according to the canon law of the Church, can be performed only by an ordained priest (or higher prelate), with the express permission of the local bishop, and only after a careful medical examination to exclude the possibility of mental illness. It seemed that the exorcism was the triggering factor moving the situation from obsession to possession, rather than the clear diagnosis of possession required before starting an exorcism. Indeed, the diagnostic criteria for demonic possession as indicated by the Roman Ritual are clear. What are these signs?

Some of the signs indicated in the Roman Ritual, as well as others suggested by the prestigious official exorcist of the Vatican, Father Gabriel Amorth, are (1999)[11]:

> The ability of the possessed to speak with some facility in a strange tongue or to understand it when spoken by another person, even when the possessed is ignorant of the language.
> The facility of the possessed in divulging future and hidden events.
> A display of powers that are beyond the subject's age and natural condition.
> Various other indications, which, when taken together as a whole, build up the evidence (p. 641).

Based on these criteria, had Father Bowdern sufficient proof to proceed with an exorcism? So far, up to the point where he got involved in the case, the evidence did not meet the criteria of the Ritual required to proceed with an exorcism, at least in terms of the first three signs above:

1. Ronald never manifested xenoglossia.
2. He did not seem to have the ability to reveal future or hidden information.
3. He did not display powers beyond his age and natural ability.

However, he seemed to have manifested some symptoms or phenomena that resembled typical poltergeist cases.

So what made the priest decide to carry out an exorcism without sufficient evidence? Did he act in an irresponsible manner and perhaps induce possession in the adolescent by introducing exorcism into the situation? According to the information evaluated so far, this does seem to be the case. Father Bowdern proceeded to begin exorcism in a case of obsession, perhaps indirectly turning it into one of possession. Furthermore, when the formal rite of exorcism started on March 18, a new series of events began, recorded by the diarist, that more resembled the symptoms of demonic possession.

These symptoms require evaluation in the light of the criteria used by the Roman Ritual, in order to determine if they qualify for a case of demonic possession. Here I will rely on the definition and criterion used by Balducci (1990), namely that one may never attribute any phenomena to preternatural causes if there is a natural cause to account for the events.

Father Bowdern, the main exorcist in the case, began the formal rite of exorcism on March 16, 1949, accompanied by his assistant Father Bishop. First, he led Ronald in an act of contrition, and then he began the prayers of exorcism according to the Roman Ritual.

Initial Sign of Demonic Possession: As Marcas do Diablo *(Diabolical Stigmata)*

One symptom that manifested intensely during the onset of the exorcism was the marks that appeared on the boy's body, apparently spontaneously. It may have been these marks that led Bowdern to conclude that this was a case of obsession, since they seemed to be attacks on the boy by the entity. According to published reports, the marks manifested at the onset of prayers; as they were being said, Ronald would wince and roll about in a seizure, with red welts appearing on his body. These were so intense that, in a rather short period of time, 25 marks appeared.

Nevertheless, it is important to realize that what may have started as a genuine dermatological problem, due to a conversion reaction, may have ended up as a case of malingering, where the adolescent may have caused some of the marks on himself to deceive his parents and the exorcists. For instance, at one point during the exorcism, one of the exorcist's assistants noticed him making the scratches on himself. As Allen has indicated in his book *Possessed*: "Robbie's right hand began moving on his chest. Van Roo looked down. Blood. He had not noticed the length of Robbie's fingernails. With one of those fingernails Robbie was scratching two words on his chest in large capital letters: HELL and Christ" (p. 161). This description clearly indicates that the boy caused some of the marks himself, which supports the hypothesis that he was malingering to some extent.

The DSM-IV defines malingering as the "intentional production of false or grossly exaggerated physical or psychological symptoms, motivated by external incentives such avoiding work" (DSM-IV-TR #V65.2). It differs from Conversion Reaction and other somatoform disorders by the intentional production of symptoms. Did Ronald have a motivation to maintain the role of being sick or possessed? The response seems to be affirmative, as in this way he could avoid attending school and would be taken to St. Louis to be with his aunt. His intrapsychic need to maintain the sick role is also suggestive of a Factious Disorder (DSM-IV, p. 683).

It must be said, however, that some of the marks seem to have appeared spontaneously, while the boy was being observed, particularly in response to the sacred words of the exorcism. For instance, in this regard Allen points out: "The exorcist immediately began the Praecipio. He had only spoken a few words when Robbie squirmed, tore open his pajamas, and revealed a scratch that was rippling along his stomach even as Bowdern and the Manheins watched" (p. 159). Also, other more dramatic marks appeared spontaneously. How can we explain these marks—if, indeed, there is a scientific explanation for them? The Jesuit priest Father Oscar González Quevedo, an international expert on demonic possession, in his book on demonic possession *Antes que os demonios voltem*[12] calls them the "marks of the Devil" or "diabolical stigmata."

Throughout history, stigmata, or "saintly marks" known as dermographia, have been interpreted by some theologians as a manifestation of divinity on the body of a saint. Often presumed to accompany religious ecstasy, they are taken as signs of holiness. Among those stigmatized saints is St. Francis of Assisi, who was said to be the first stigmatic in Christian history. Of the more than 330 persons identified with stigmata since the 14th century, more than 60 have been canonized or beatified by the Roman Catholic Church. According to contemporary biographers of St. Francis, he manifested in his later life wounds on his hands, his feet, and his side, which bled profusely and were intensely painful. St. Catherine of Siena reputedly bore invisible stigmata, which became visible after her death. The Roman Catholic Church investigates every such instance, but avoids any pronouncement on their nature or cause. Modern stigmatics (including in the 20th-century Therese Neumann and the Capuchin Padre Pio) have been examined by scientific medical authorities, who are inclined to believe that the stigmata are connected with nervous or cataleptic hysteria.

Obviously, if we posit the existence of saintly stigmata, the opposite is diabolical stigmata, being signs of the Devil, who opposes God. Therefore, the presence of diabolical stigmata is an expected sign of diabolical manifestation in cases of possession. Father Quevedo[13] points out that these diabolical marks were branded on the bodies or witches in sexual orgies with demonic succubi or incubi; thus these sexual demons would make marks on the bodies of witches by sucking on them. These are the explanations, he added, offered by the *Malleus Malleficarium* for the marks on witches made by the demons. Consequently, the presence of diabolical stigmata has meaning opposite to that of saintly stigmata.

In conclusion, even though some of these marks are hard to explain by science, most scientists and dermatological experts agree that there are a number of medical conditions that could account for this disorder. Thus, regarding the Mount Rainier incident, Quevedo explains the mark reading "Help me" that appeared on the body of the possessed girl (in the fictionalized version by Blatty) as follows: "The dermographic marks that appeared on her stomach reading 'Help me'—it was not the demon who was asking for help, but the poor possessed woman [*sic*], who was painfully stranded and had her hands tied to the bed and could not ask for help. This nervous tension of being tied up to the bed led to somatization to ask via her body for help since she could not write or move her hands to ask for help" (173).

What explains stigmatization? Is it Jesus reminding us through His messengers of the pain He suffered as He redeemed mankind? Is it a biological process tied to religious mentational activity—the biotheological phenomenon par excellence? Or is it simply fraud, whether intentional or not?

We know that emotions can cause skin eruptions. The medical term for this is psychogenic purpuras, bruising and bleeding from the skin from emotional stress. However, these look like bruises, or spots—not wounds. And the bleeding is subdural—under the skin (Fierro, 2006).[14]

There are substantial grounds for doubting supernatural explanations, besides the fact that some stigmatics themselves have admitted that they were frauds (such as Magdalena de la Cruz, 1487–1560). There is no video or other objective, scientific account of a stigmatic episode. It seems suspicious that stigmatization would have emerged in the 1200s, right when there was an emphasis on the Crucifixion, and then largely died out over the last few hundred years. Furthermore, stigmata ordinarily appear on people's palms, whereas it now seems likely that the actual wounds were in Jesus' wrists. Virtually all stigmatics are Roman Catholic.

Stepping back, we see that the relationship between the corporeal and the divine is one of the most complex and profound in our psychosocial spaces. Clearly, the physical body is our vehicle for experiencing the Ultimate and its gift to us. It is not surprising that we would find intriguing phenomena at this boundary, or that world religions mark and celebrate it with ceremonies and rituals involving the body, including flagellation—not to mention circumcision.

Ian Wilson, author of *The Bleeding Mind: An Investigation into the Mysterious Phenomenon of Stigmata*,[15] believes that stigmata are a manifestation of undiscovered abilities of the mind to influence the very shape and functioning of the human body, related to the supposed ability to heal warts with your mind (or increase your breast size). According to Wilson, the "phenomenon is a psychological one, with a pathology related closely to multiple personality disorder. Stress and poverty in early life are a common thread running through the lives of many stigmatists. Nearly all suffered some sort of personal catastrophe before the onset of the stigmata, and nearly all had a predisposition to trance states and other altered modes of consciousness. Apparently stigmatists identify so closely with the life of Christ and visualize Him so clearly that some undiscovered physiological mechanism imposes Christ's marks of suffering on the body of the stigmatist" (p. 164).

Can we explain by the same mechanism the diabolical stigmata of the Mount Rainier case? It seems that there is enough ground to explain these demonic stigmata by natural mechanisms of the brain, under very special psychological conditions, that science can fully explain in most cases. What we know about dermatology at the present time leads us to conclude that it would be hard to take the marks as convincing signs of possession, since we would first have to rule out all natural causes after a careful medical evaluation by a dermatologist. Otherwise, no matter what kind of marks appeared, spontaneous or not spontaneous, they would first have to be evaluated by an expert, not taken for granted as an absolute sign of possession. Indeed, this was the attitude of the careful Lutheran minister who initially evaluated the case; thus, in one of his letters he states: "My physician saw no marks, they seemed to be more like nervous rashes."[16] His insistence that medical experts evaluate the adolescent first resulted in his being ousted from the case by a family unhappy with his scientific approach. As he expressed in a later interview, "I have no doubt that the family did not like the way I handled matters with Ronald and decided to cut me off from the case; they wanted to find somebody who would conform to the expectations of their beliefs on the case."[17]

Based on the information available on the Mount Rainier case, we can infer that the initial marks that appeared on the boy's body seem to have been made by him; however, as his condition worsened, his psychological tension may have ended up being expressed in actual marks that were the result of the somatization of the stress he was undergoing. It seems that the introduction of the exorcism aggravated the symptoms to the point where new phenomena conformed more to actual cases of demonic possession.

We can thus identify two periods of marks on the boy's body, the first being those appearing prior to the introduction of the exorcism, which had these very interesting features:

First, they appeared mostly in the absence of witnesses, when the boy was by himself and near the bathroom or in his private room where sharp objects were sometimes kept, or where he could maneuver freely by himself. The modus operandi following the appearance of these marks was that he would yell for help, causing a family member to dash upstairs to see the marks already present on his body under his pajamas.

Secondly, the marks were ordinarily reported by the adolescent to the family members and later to the priest. They were mostly connected with the boy's wish to avoid going to school. For instance, large marks in the form of the letter "N" branded his body whenever his mother raised the issue of school. When his desire to go to St. Louis where his favorite aunt lived came into play, the marks even indicated the location and the day and time of departure, as in marks reading "St. Louis," "Saturday," and "3½ weeks."

Interestingly, most of the aforementioned characteristics related to the diagnosis of conversion reaction mentioned above in the context of his psychological evaluation.

Next, we have the marks that appeared after the exorcism was introduced. Now the theme changes to being more related to demonic possession, or what we have called diabolical stigmata. Among the features of the marks are these:

> They increase in frequency as the exorcism becomes more intense.
> They are more related to demonic subject matter, featuring marks such as "Hell."
> They appear spontaneously, with more complex letters and images on the skin, and with witnesses present
> The marks appear in response to the exorcism being performed

At one point in this progression, a dermatologist was consulted on the possible origins of such marks and figures as the red welts forming an image of a bat on the boy's leg (as described by Bishop on p. 94 of *Possessed*), or others in the form of letters that could actually be read on his skin. Bishop described these in the following terms: the "marks rise up above the surface of the skin, similar to an engraving" (p. 93).

Regarding the above description of the marks, the dermatologist who was consulted indicated, "the appearance of marks that rise up on the surface of the skin, spontaneously on the skin of a person, is a condition which may be present in people who undergo or confront severe stress and the stress affects the skin via a somatization of it. However, the formation of spontaneous letters and complicated images such as in this case, would be hard to explain via normal dermatological conditions that we know of in our field."

Nevertheless, there are other cases in the history of spontaneous marks or diabolical stigmata that could shed light into the spontaneous marks that appeared spontaneously on the adolescent body in the view of his parents and the exorcist. For instance, Father Quevedo relates the historical case of Mother Jeanne des Anges, the main diabolically possessed person of the witches of Loudun. Quevedo points out, "During the last session of exorcism, suddenly she yelled and afterwards she expressed loudly a name, Jose [Joseph]. We all turned around and saw on her raised forearm a spontaneous mark emerging in red blood. We examined the mark and noticed that it was the name Jose engraved in her forearm measuring about 3 centimeters" (p. 172).

Samsonism: Vires Supra Natura *(Force Beyond Your Nature)*

Another sign indicated by the Ritual is referred by father Quevedo as Samsonism (referring to the biblical story of Samson in Judges 13–16, about a man who was given great strength by God). Superhuman strength is considered by the Roman Ritual as one of the main signs of demonic possession. According to Thomas Allen, the manifestation of superhuman strength by the adolescent would support the case in favor of demonic possession. In the movie *The Exorcist*, Linda Blair displayed superhuman strength when she threw the director of her mother's movie out of a window; he appeared later under the balcony with his head turned completely backwards.

Historically, in the Bible we can trace the first manifestation of superhuman strength as part of demonic possession in the Gadarene story in the New Testament. The Bible describes the event: "Then they sailed to the country of the Gadarenes, which is opposite Galilee. And when He stepped out on the land, there met Him a certain man from the city who had demons for a long time. And he wore no clothes, nor did he live in a house but in the tombs.... For it had often seized him, and he was kept under guard, bound with chains and shackles; and he broke the bonds and was driven by the demon into the wilderness" (Luke 8:26–27, 29). Some biblical theologians have interpreted this story as a man who was possessed by the devil, as a result of which he manifested superhuman strength. This account is the apparent source of the acceptance of superhuman strength as a sign of possession. The Ritual includes it as one of its symptoms.

In the Mount Rainier case, Allen provides accounts that seem to indicate that this symptom was one of those manifested by the boy:

[A]t Christina dominium, Robbie thrashed more violently. Bowdern signaled Halloran to come around the bed and hold Robbie down. Halloran, a strapping athlete, could not hold down the ninety-five-pound boy (p. 96).

Bowdern opened the Ritual again and the three Jesuits resumed the chant of the litany.... Robbie erupted, arms, legs flailing. He tore at the blanket and sheet, pummeled the pillow. Halloran moved to the head of the bed and grabbed the boy. His father and uncle rushed in and joined Halloran. All three of the men were holding Robbie down. Yet he twisted and arched his body. The contortions, Bishop later recorded, "revealed physical strength beyond the natural power of Robbie" (p. 110).

According to some reports on the case, as many as ten people were needed to hold him down as a result of the powerful strength he was able to manifest. This, however, seems to be a gross exaggeration, and makes us wonder about the physical space needed in order even to touch the boy, let alone hold him down. How did all those people manage even to get close to the boy in the small physical space where the exorcism was taking place? Unless they resorted to some kind of special arrangement giving them space to maneuver, it would be almost impossible to get 10 people to touch a body simultaneously, particularly the body of a 95-pound youngster.

The Roman Ritual is very subjective in its discussion of this sign, since it does not provide parameters to determine what constitutes superhuman strength. Do the possessed, for example, have to manifest the ability to carry or lift a certain number of pounds? Or does the possessed have to be able to perform incredible feats of strength? How can this be determined in the context of a very subjective ambience, charged with emotional turmoil for the exorcist and his assistants?

It is important to note that reports on the Mount Rainier case vary. For instance, in his detailed account, Thomas Allen set the number at three persons needed to hold the boy down, while other reports on the case, such as one that appeared in the *National Tattler* (1974),[18] set the number at five. In his book on the case against possession, Juan Cortes used the number ten.

Consequently, it is hard to determine the real number of people required to hold down the adolescent during his seizures. Moreover, it seems that the authors relied on a subjective sense of the supposedly superhuman strength demonstrated by Ronald as reported and perceived by Halloran. For instance, he considered that the boy's ability to "twist and arch his body" while being held down by three people indicated that he had superhuman strength beyond his natural capacity.[19]

In the Mount Rainier case, in any event, we do not see anything like the superhuman strength portrayed in the film of *The Exorcist*, that ends up with somebody being thrown out a window with his head twisted all the way backwards. We see something more like what happens in some mental wards, where inmates may have to be held down by two or three people when they are in crisis. I have seen even some younger patients in a pediatrician's office who had to be held down by the doctor, a relative and/or a nurse when they were supposed to be taking injections or medications. These children, even while being held down, are able to twist and arch their bodies, but this does not necessarily mean that they possess superhuman strength!

We do have in history some cases where clear signs of superhuman strength have been demonstrated, and where the decision to diagnose this activity as one of possession is more credible. In his book titled *Possession*,[20] Oesterreich writes: "[T]he affective disorder of the possessed is translated by their movements, which equal in intensity those of veritable raving madmen. It must, however, be added that these movements cannot be entirely resolved into expressions of emotions and their derived manifestations, a great number appearing to come from an autonomous excitement of the motor system. For the movements are particularly deprived of sense."

For instance, he cites the following case: "When Durr began his magnetic [hypnotic] manipulations, the whole body twisted and reared with such ease and rapidity that one may have believed it under the dominance of an external force ... quickly he [the supposed demon of the patient] rose with such violence that she sat up on the sofa when it was least expected and could not be forced to lie down again in spite of the aid of five persons present, mostly strong men" (p. 23). In this case, we see elements that seem to be more suggestive of superhuman strength beyond the natural age of the possessed than in the Mount Rainier case. This was an instance of a fragile and sick woman who was able to evidence such strength, even to the point of almost strangling one of the exorcist's assistants.

The subjective nature of the symptom of superhuman strength as a sign of possession led Rodewyk (1974)[21] to broaden its scope. In this regard he wrote: "In speaking of 'extraordinary powers' we have the tendency to concentrate on the purely bodily and physical side of such phenomena. But the psychological or psychic feats ... belong to this category" (p. 92). Thus in his extended definition of superhuman strength, indicated in the Roman Ritual as Powers that are beyond person's age or natural condition, the author presents the following symptoms as complementary: precognition, levitation, unusual weight, hypnotic states, psychosomatic illnesses such as sudden appearance of marks on the skin, and other related symptoms.[22]

Regarding the aforementioned symptoms, it is important to note that they are not present in the Mount Rainier case; there are no instances of levitation, even though one of the members of the circle of prayers declared that there was some levitation during the prayers performed by friends of the family in the house of the adolescent. In another instance, there were reports that levitation occurred at some point during the exorcism. Nevertheless, these are merely informal reports that do not appear in the formal record. Moreover, there are no instances of a display of precognition or telepathy on the part of the possessed. Such signs, as indicated by Rodewyk, would certainly have reinforced the argument for possession in the Mount Rainier case.

Regarding his complementary signs, Rodewyk recognizes, however, that the aforementioned symptoms are unique and may or not may be observed in specific possession cases. Moreover, he indicates, they could be found in some categories of psychic phenomena currently under investigation in the areas of psychology and parapsychology. In other words, the aforementioned phenomena could be explained by psychological and parapsychological mechanisms and thus are not necessarily indicative of demonic possession.

Furthermore, in the determination of cases that are genuine in nature as demonic possession versus others that may be explained by natural causes, Rodewyk follows the path of Balducci, suggesting the need to "look for specific tonality observed in manic episodes and certain psychiatric conditions (e.g., catatonia does not show normal fatigue)" (Bufford, 1989; Quevedo, 1989).[23]

As Quevedo has pointed out, "Samsonism or superhuman strength can ... appear under hypnosis, trance, hysteria and in some neuroses and psychoses, with absolute variety and totally independent of a religious connotation ... that is enough to understand that we are dealing with a human phenomenon" (1989, p. 124).

The term Samsonism is used by Quevedo to refer to the Biblical story of Samson and Delilah, where Samson had acquired superhuman strength due to his long hair as a form of divine power. We can conclude from the aforementioned information that the "superhuman strength" shown by the possessed may just be normal strength "enhanced" in an altered state of consciousness experienced by the participants. Recently, a patient related to me that at some point in his life he had witnessed an incredible feat of strength by his mother, who was able to pull his son out from under a heavy piece of metal that had fallen on him. The piece of metal was so heavy that the patient himself was later unable to lift it, even though under the immediately terrible circumstances of the accident she had been able to save the boy's life.

It is important to note that stress causes the body to produce chemical substances that increase our physical strength under the so-called fight-or-flight response. This means that, when we are in danger or in a fight, we may experience a cascade of hormones that trigger our body to respond with a strength that under normal circumstances would not be available to us.

Furthermore, it is important to note that superhuman strength has been found in people under altered states of consciousness such as trance or hypnosis. It is known that possession also constitutes a state of trance, one that produces somnambulistic or hypnotic states (Sargant, 1974).[24] In support of this hypothesis, Sargant has argued that there are similarities between possession and somnambulistic states, in support of which position he points to Oesterreich's (1966)[25] definition of possession as a state of somnambulism, although with some differences: "A state in which normal individuality is temporarily replaced by another and which leaves no memory on return to the normal, must be called according to present terminology, one of somnambulism. Typical possession is nevertheless distinguished from ordinary somnambulistic states by its intense and emotional excitement" (p. 39).

Xenoglossy: Ignota Lingua Loqui (*Speaking Unknown Languages*)

There is another sign of possession, as indicated by the Roman Ritual, known as xenoglossy, which may be explained by the aforementioned mechanism suggested by Sargant (1974). Xenoglossy, one of the signs of demonic possession according to the Roman Ritual, is the ability to speak or understand a foreign language never previously studied. According to the Italian researcher on the paranormal Ernesto Bozzano, in his publication *Mediumnidad Poliglota* (Multilingual Mediumship), xenoglossy is the greatest real proof of communication between the dead and living humans.

In the Mount Rainier case, there is no indication, at least in the more serious or formal reports such as the diary in Allen's detailed analysis, that Ronald was able to speak or understand a language that he had never studied. There were, however, popular reports in the media suggesting that he was able to do so.

For instance, in the initial report of the case that appeared in the *Washington Post* (August 20, 1949, 1A),[26] the author Bill Brinkley reported: "[T]he boy broke into a violent tantrum of screaming, cursing and voicing of Latin phrases—a language he had never studied—whenever the priest reached the climatic point of the Ritual." Moreover, according to O'Leary of the *Washington Star-News* (1973),[27] the boy was also able to speak in a language resembling modern Hebrew; according to a professor of Oriental languages who was invited to see the boy, he recognized the language as Aramaic, a language spoken in Palestine in Jesus' times.

When I asked the Reverend Schulze in the course of our personal interview if he was familiar with any reports of xenoglossy on the part of the boy, he said that the Jesuits' reports to which he had access never mentioned such phenomena, nor was there any information offered by the family to him of xenoglossy. However, even if the reports of xenoglossy in the popular media were correct, there is a mental mechanism that can account for it. For instance, Sargant (1974) has argued that xenoglossy may be explained by a process in which the brain absorbs and records far more information than is normally remembered, but which can come to the surface in abnormal states of mind. In explaining the phenomenon, he states: "It has never been satisfactorily proved that anyone has spoken a foreign language with they had no previous acquaintance, and while proving a negative is rationally difficult, we do know that people in hypnotic states can sometimes remember foreign words and phrases which they learned in the past but have forgotten. In their suggestible state they may well come to believe that they are speaking in tongues and they may easily convey this conviction to others around them who are equally uncritical because the whole group is in a high state of suggestibility" (p. 27).

Interestingly, this group mechanism of suggestibility indicates that Sargant could actually be explaining why other members of a group may become so credulous when the phenomenon is one that they all are experiencing at the same time. It is well known that some religious leaders, such as David Koresh and other ministers, have used altered states of consciousness similar to hypnosis in order to convey their messages; in some cases, they have even led members to commit suicide in the name of God. Since hypnosis facilitates suggestibility in a person, a similar effect may be created via prayers, which are sometimes carried out in a much-altered state of mind in the context of religious chants. These mechanisms may facilitate group suggestibility, similar to what takes place in an exorcism, which plays out in the context of a group experiencing an altered state of consciousness via the prayers and the forcible casting out of demons. In such a context, what may be a normal manifestation of physical strength by the "possessed" may, due to the subject's altered state of consciousness, be misinterpreted by those around as superhuman strength.

The following case, which I experienced as a member of the Pentecostal Church, may illustrate the above point. In 1982, during a Circle of Prayer organized at a private home by members of my church and myself, a young adolescent of about fifteen, while the prayers were being said, began suddenly to speak in what Pentecostals call tongues. This young woman was known by some members of the church who were present as a person "baptized by the Holy Spirit" and possessing the special spiritual gift of being able to speak in tongues.

At one of these prayer sessions, she indeed began to speak in tongues. Coincidentally, I had invited to this session a friend of mine who was fluent in German; to his surprise, he recognized the language she was speaking while in some sort of trance as German. He then carefully transcribed the German phrases she was uttering. After the prayer session, my friend commented that the phrases, while actual German utterances, were loose expressions without a sequence, more as if she were reading structured phrases out of a book on literature—that is, they were related but not connected.

When questioned about her knowledge of German, the girl denied any familiarity with the language. Nevertheless, further investigation among other family members revealed that at one point in her life, she had a friend who had been born in Germany who used to teach her basic, unconnected German phrases.

As Sargant (1974) has pointed out, a state of trance combined with heightened susceptibility triggers recall of material stored in long-term memory. It is perfectly plausible that pieces of information that arise from this trance-like state may take the form of loose phrases from languages not well learned and apparently forgotten. The Jesuit priest Father Oscar Gonzalez Quevedo, in his book *El rostro oculto de la mente* (The Occult Side of the Mind), called this mechanism pantomnesia (from the Greek pantos, meaning all, and mnemos, meaning memory).[28] According to Quevedo, we never forget most stimuli to which we are exposed during our conscious life, but they are stored in the long-term memory from where they may arise during altered states of consciousness such as hypnosis or possession. Therefore, a language we once learned, or phrases of a language, may be apparently forgotten, but during a trance may return to the conscious level.

In sum, I believe that most cases of xenoglossy or glossolalia, particularly those that take place during the altered states of consciousness of possession and religious prayer, may be explained by the aforementioned mechanisms. A similar view has been expressed by other authors such as Quevedo (1974),[29] Heredia (1922),[30] and Richet (1923).[31] Moreover, Quevedo has raised the question as to why the devil would be interested in speaking in a particular foreign language. And if so, when interrogated in another language, why is he not able to respond? As a superior supernatural force, it would not be hard for him to answer when interrogated in a language other than the one he is speaking through the possessed.

Quevedo[32] also points to the case of Annelise Mitchell, who was exorcised by the missionary Father Arnold Rens during the fifteen years he spent in China. During the exorcism, it occurred to him to interrogate the demon in Chinese. In response, the possessed replied, "If you wish to speak to me, it has to be in German." Quevedo adds, "It would be also contradictory that the demon would not be able to maintain a conversation at a level superior to the knowledge of Annelise."

15

The Final Questions

As the reader skims through the pages of this book, questions will inevitably arise regarding *The Exorcist* and the Mount Rainier case on which it was based. To respond to some of these questions, I have decided to use a question-response format to aid in understanding those questions considered seminal in the proposal of this book and that would provide a better glimpse of the case to the reader.

Among these questions are the following: Before you read this book, were you a believer or nonbeliever in demonic possession? Were the witnesses of these cases victims of collective suggestion that led them to see things that were not actually there? How reliable and truthful are the documents such as the Jesuit Diary, also known as the Jesuit Report, in relating the events surrounding the Mount Rainier case? What happened to the family after the exorcism was over? Was Ronald really possessed by the Devil?

However, before responding to these questions, I will address the perennial debate of two groups, which over the years have been attempting to prove or disprove the existence of the supernatural by any and all means. Both groups have been determined to prove their point no matter what evidence supports or refutes a case, such as the Mount Rainier Exorcism. In this scientific/religious dispute, the Mount Rainier case and *The Exorcist* have been used by believers in demonic possession to try to prove the case is authentic, or used by skeptics to disprove demonic possession and exorcism. Unfortunately, both sides of this controversy hold preconceived beliefs committed to proving or disproving the supernatural, many times independently of the evidence presented to them in favor or against. Such biases compromise the position of any researcher who investigates these types of cases in attempting to reach the scientific truth independently of supernatural or atheistic beliefs.

Moreover, the premises held by the aforementioned groups have been utilized by previous writers on the Mount Rainier case and *The Exorcist*, in their writings (in popular as well as scientific forums) in trying to prove a point instead of pursuing scientific validity and serving the public for whom the issues of demonic possession and exorcism are serious matters in the context of their faith.

Consequently, these writers have at times ignored evidence that would support the opposite group's position. In my opinion, any writer has the responsibility to convey the truth to his/her readers independently of his/her own personal beliefs. However, most previous writers on these matters were trying to protect their personal religious faith or scientific orientation in spite of evidence contrary to their prejudiced beliefs.

Some pertinent questions related to *The Exorcist* and the Mount Rainier case:

Question 1: *Were you a believer ("sheep") in the existence of demonic possession and exorcism, or a nonbeliever ("goat"), before reading this book? Before providing an answer, consider the concept of the sheep–goat effect that I have borrowed from experimental parapsychological research. Also, as previously mentioned in this book, in some parapsychological experiments, people who believe in extrasensory perception (sheep) tend to score above chance, while those who do not believe in extrasensory perception (goats) show null results or psi-missing (significantly worse than chance performance) on a psi test. This has become known as the "sheep–goat effect."*

Response: Nonbelievers (goats) and some researchers of demonic possession and exorcism hold the premise, "If you believe in the devil you will see the devil in *The Exorcist* and the Mount Rainier case, even if the devil isn't there." However, according to this view, if you do not see demonic possession in the Mount Rainier case, it follows that you don't believe in the devil. In other words, the suggestibility factor or personal belief system may be responsible for whether or not you see the devil in demonic possession cases such as the Mount Rainier Exorcism. I believe that most previous writers and researchers on *The Exorcist* and the Mount Rainier case fall into one of two categories. Among them, John Nicola, in his book *Diabolical Possession*, and Thomas Allen, author of *Possessed*, fall into the believer's religious category, along with the priests and family members of the Hunkeler family who participated in the case. They have interpreted the facts and ostensible paranormal events that took place in the Mount Rainier case as demonic possession events according to their religious belief system; in other words, they drew their conclusions based on what they believed or wanted to believe.

The aforementioned people held religious views that predisposed them to believe that the events surrounding the Mount Rainier case were entirely valid and true. Other experts with a more skeptical orientation, such as atheists or certain writers of the *Skeptical Enquirer*, would say that this case is fraudulent or could be explained by natural, scientific mechanisms, no matter what appearances or the evidence may suggest.

The problem with this type of individual, whether believer or nonbeliever, is that they have embraced their belief system as part of a dogma to defend, which hardly serves scientific inquiry or the general public when considering cases of ostensible supernatural or paranormal phenomena.

Perhaps the most objective and scientific position regarding the Mount Rainier case, in spite of his religious orientation, was held by the Lutheran Rev. Luther Miles Schulze, who maintained a cautious position and tried to explain the case by science, but with an open mind to other possible hypotheses and explanations. This is the most interesting position pertaining to the case, particularly coming from a serious witness with a firsthand account of the events.

The Rev. Luther Miles Schulze was never credulous about the events declared to him to be true by the family of the allegedly possessed adolescent boy. When describing the paranormal events reported by the family, but that he did not himself witness, Schulze distanced himself and often used the phrase "the family tells me…."[1] He even tried to demonstrate that a healer invited by the family to help Ronald was a fake. However, when he conducted an experiment to prove that the boy was not subject to demonic possession and persisted in his intent to follow up with a scientific approach, the family then removed him from the case.

Moreover, in explaining the marks that appeared on the boy's body, he declared in a letter to renowned parapsychologist J.B. Rhine that he saw no such marks but did see some nerve rashes.[2] However, he was shocked by what he had witnessed the night the boy spent at his premises. Up to the time when I interviewed the Rev. Luther Miles Schulze in 1993, he declared, "The boy was not faking it…. I wonder if I was going screwy."[3]

In spite of what he had witnessed, Schulze did not rely on demonic possession to explain the phenomena, and in the years after I initially interviewed him, he has maintained this position. Instead, he tried to put Ronald into the hands of professionals familiar with the phenomena, such as Dr. J.B. Rhine, and also took the boy to see his personal medical doctor.

Consequently, I believe the Reverend Schulze is the witness with the most objective approach in the Mount Rainier case, which leads us to the possibility that some of the phenomena in the case may have been genuine, since he was a nonbeliever, unlikely to be deceived by suggestibility. Nonetheless, he still witnessed phenomena that he could not explain, in spite of the possibility that Ronald may have deceived him. However, the kind of phenomena that he witnessed was so compelling that it is hard to believe that he was entirely deceived by the adolescent boy. His testimony is only suggestive of ostensible paranormal phenomena that may have taken place and that he could not explain.

In my view, it is better to be critical of any phenomenon rather than to dismiss it out of hand, regardless of my own belief system, so that I do not deceive myself with personal beliefs, even more so in investigating such a prominent case in the history of demonology. This is a difficult position to maintain; however, it is the most useful for a reader of this book to consider the facts with an open mind.

Question 2: Is it possible to assess the Mount Rainier case scientifically after all the time that has passed since it took place?

Response: First of all, the facts that are used to investigate the events surrounding the Mount Rainier Exorcism would have to be accurate and truthful. Regarding the accuracy of the events, as related in the Jesuit Report, and from the witnesses and religious members involved, it is important to note that the case took place over a half century ago. Consequently, it is difficult to assess the accuracy of the facts as though the case had taken place more recently or in the present. Nevertheless, we now have information never before released about the events surrounding the Mount Rainier Exorcism that will make it much easier to evaluate this case at the present time.

Question 3: Are the documents that previous writers have relied on to assess the Mount Rainier case reliable or genuine regarding the account of the events?

Response: There are a couple of written sources regarding the Mount Rainier Exorcism that I want to address here, the first and perhaps most famous of which is the Jesuit's Diary or Jesuit Report. This document was apparently found in the Alexian Brothers Hospital in St. Louis and was written by one of the priests who participated in the exorcism. Thomas B. Allen, author of the book *Possessed*, apparently obtained a copy of the Diary, which consists of approximately 20 pages of entries. I had access to a comparable document at the Foundation for Research on the Nature of Man with contents similar to those of the Diary, which the Reverend Schulze named the "Jesuit Document."

Also, when I interviewed Luther Schulze, he asked his assistant of many years, Ida Mae, to provide me with a copy of the Jesuit Report that she had kept for the records of the Lutheran Church. In addition, a copy was sent to the Lutheran Synod in Washington, D.C., by the Reverend Schulze in 1949. The Jesuit Report constitutes a daily report of all the events that took place during the second exorcism. However, the account of the Diary regarding the events during the exorcism was written by a credulous priest, who accepted as facts what he had been told by the family and reported them as such with an unquestioning mind. Therefore, the priests were sheep (believers in demonic possession).

The second source, the one I consider the most reliable on the Mount Rainier Exorcism, is the extensive correspondence between the Rev. Luther Schulze and Dr. J.B. Rhine. Also significant is the report of events that he sent to Dr. Rhine at Duke University and to Dick Darnell, the president of the Parapsychology Society in Washington, back in 1949. I believe these last two documents are the most reliable sources we have on the case since they were written by an outsider, who really wanted to get to the bottom of this case. Also, the Reverend Schulze followed a very scientific approach to investigate it, particularly when he pressed the family to take their son to a doctor for a medical evaluation.

Also, when he suspected that some events were taking place could not be explained by normal explanations, he then contacted Dr. J.B. Rhine at Duke University Parapsychology Laboratory. Interestingly, Rhine provided the Reverend Schulze with some guidance as to how to investigate the case in an objective manner. Schulze, in one of his letters to Rhine, insisted that a competent person, sympathetic to the case, could investigate it, and even suggested that if Rhine or one of his staff members could not investigate the case, then someone from Harvard University. Not only did he not try to provide an explanation for the events, but his attitude shows that he wanted this case to be investigated by experts in the area of medicine and psychology.

I would conclude, in response to the question at hand, that documents such as the Jesuit Diary are more reliable in terms of describing the events, as they took place during the actual exorcism. However, the Diary or Jesuit Report is not as reliable regarding the objective perception of the events themselves. It is important to note that the diarist, who witnessed the events under an altered state of consciousness, may have been deceived either by trickery or the emotional state under which he wrote the story, leading him to record things that were not true. Moreover, it is important to note that he witnessed the events under a high level of stress and suggestibility, mental states which may have influenced his perception of the events. However, the letters seem to be a more reliable source of the events since they were written by a nonbeliever with a guarded position, and with a scientific approach in mind.

Question 4: Did suggestibility play a factor in deceiving the witnesses of this case?

Response: Yes, in my opinion most of the events in the Mount Rainier case took place under uncontrolled, spontaneously unexpected conditions, and seem to have caught many of the original witnesses of the case by surprise. The supposedly paranormal events that took place in the Mount Rainier Exorcism were events that occurred with people under altered states of consciousness and under heightened stress, states that may have facilitated the suggestibility of the participants to see things that were not there. This is why in a certain part of their correspondence, J.B. Rhine warns the Rev. Luther Schulz about the ostensible paranormal events he had witnessed and asks whether or not they were observed under good lighting.

Under an "altered state of consciousness," people can perceive events that are not real but that are the product of their mind's suggestibility. In this regard, I will relate a personal experience during an experiment conducted at the university where I trained as a specialist in hypnosis. One of my professors, an expert in clinical hypnosis, conducted an experiment of group suggestibility. During one of his lectures, suddenly he stepped out of the classroom and returned a few minutes later, agitated and yelling that the laboratory where monkeys where housed for experiments was on fire. All of us rushed out of the building, and then he yelled at us again, telling us that the monkeys from the laboratory were on the top of the roof of the psychology building trying to escape the fire. Most of the students, including myself, looked at the top of the roof of the building and actually saw the monkeys trying to escape. Minutes later he laughed at us and told us, "There are no monkeys in the roof; this is just your imagination ... an experiment of suggestibility." This collective suggestibility experiment actually worked.

My personal view is that some of the participants, even those acting in good faith such as the Reverend Schulze, may have been caught off guard with the unexpected events that occurred with and around the boy. This was indicated to the Rev. Luther Schulze by J.B. Rhine in a letter dated April 21, 1949, who warned him, "The reason I take this guarded position is that a number of these cases have been reduced to clever trickery, and since we are not ordinarily prepared for the unusual sort (rather pathological) of faking that is sometimes practiced, we are not as guarded as would be required to see everything that is going on in such cases."[4]

Question 5: *What happened to Ronald Hunkeler and his family after the exorcism was over?*

Response: When I visited Ida Mae Donley, a close friend of the family, for a second interview back in 1993, although the Hunkeler family had moved out of the area, they continued to be in contact with her in Mount Rainier. During our conversation that afternoon, she put me on the phone with Ronald Hunkeler, but he refused to talk about the case. What I have learned about what happened shortly after the exorcism was over comes mostly from the correspondence maintained by Dick Darnell, the president of the Society for Parapsychology in Washington back in the 1940s. In a letter dated May 17, 1949, we learn that the real name of Ronald (the name used by the Reverend Schulze in his letters for the 14-year-old adolescent) was Ronald Hunkeler.[5] Also in a letter dated April 6, 1949, addressed to Dr. J.B. Rhine by the Rev. Luther Schulze, we learn that after the exorcism in St. Louis, the family returned to Prince George's County, where they lived. In this letter, the Reverend Schulze indicates that "the boy appears perfectly healthy despite the three months of antics with loss of sleep. The Jesuits here want to place him in a monastery and hold services for 21 days." According to the Reverend Schulze, they returned back home from St. Louis on April 6, 1949.[6]

Moreover, we now know that the family had no plan for what they wanted to do after the exorcism. As conveyed by the Reverend Schulze in a letter addressed to Dr. J.B. Rhine: "I wish I could give you some definite plan now as to what the family wishes to do now. Perhaps I can later." Interestingly, the Reverend Schulze learned directly from the family that now that their son was freed from the devil via the exorcism practiced by the Jesuits, "They did not want to know anything about somebody from a university," as he expressed in the letter. "They are a bit skeptical about anyone from a university, especially a psychiatrist! They feel this is entirely a religious problem" (letter dated March 21, 1949).[7]

Furthermore, while the family was in St. Louis, there was an incident in which a relative who attended Washington University "brought someone from the faculty to the house, who told them of his fantasies concerning the spirit world; that someday we could tune in to any of the departed we wished to, just as we now tune in a television program." The Reverend Schulze further explained that "the Jesuits admitted that it was the devil and finally had a service of exorcism."[8] It is important to note that the Jesuits provided a copy of the diary to the family, a copy that they shared with the Reverend Schulze.

Additionally, the Rev. Luther Schulze indicated that the family had returned, accompanied by two Jesuit priests who tried to place the recovered adolescent in a hospital, and claimed they could find no place in the area. Therefore, in a letter dated April 19, 1949, they proposed that the family to return to St. Louis in order to place Ronald in one of their hospitals again. The family appears to have had great confidence in the Catholic ritual and the priests' tales of experiences in exorcism rites.[9]

In the same letter, the Reverend Schulze expressed his concerns about the family's mental well-being. He adds, "I have a feeling that the family will require treatment as individuals and as a family and eventually they will pick up the pieces."[10] In a final note, he indicates that the boy slept that night, so he returned to the priests' rectory. At the end of this letter, Schulze reveals the two addresses where the Hunkelers lived while the exorcism and the events took place.[11]

Mr. Edwin C. Hunkeler
c/o L.C. Hunkeler
8435 Roanoke Drive
Normandy, Missouri

Mr. Edwin C. Hunkeler
3807 40th Drive
Cottage City, Maryland

Additionally, in a letter dated September 19, 1949,[12] the Reverend Schulze provides further information on the well-being of Ronald Hunkeler: "In the case that I reported, it may be of interest to you that I saw the boy in June. He had grown taller, gained weight, his neck thickened and his voice deepened. I have an idea that medical examinations would show that he reached puberty during this experience. The family is still in fear of recurrence and was quite distressed about the newspaper publicity even though their identity was concealed."

The information regarding the well-being of Ronald was complemented by Dick Darnell, president of the Society, who in a letter dated May 12, 1949, indicated to Dr. Rhine that morning, "I talked with Ronald's mother. Ronald is apparently all right now except that he talks in his sleep which probably has little or no relationship to the other. The mother had an attack of nerves and is taking medicine prescribed by the corner druggist. Ronald is still out of school but is planning to go back to summer school."

Finally, regarding the report on the case prepared by the Reverend Schulze for Dr. Rhine, Dick Darnell further indicates in a letter dated June 7, 1949: "My reason in writing is to say that I talked to Luther Schulze yesterday and he has promised to get busy on the report next week. Ronald is still apparently okay. The family incidentally has a report from the Jesuits which he will get copied for us. They stated that they would not guarantee the non-recurrence unless the family becomes Jesuit!"[13]

It is important to note that the Jesuit Report, the same document known as the Diary, was sent to J.B. Rhine at Duke University, who used it along with the one prepared by the Reverend Schulze to publish part of the case in the *Parapsychology Bulletin*. This is as far as the information on Ronald and the Hunkeler family goes in this series of letters between the Reverend Schulze, J.B. Rhine, and Dick Darnell. After this information was released in 1949, there has been no additional information on the records about what happened to the family. As a final note, I would add that this case was investigated by the Society for Parapsychology in Washington, D.C., whose researchers provided the means to write the report, such as the stenographer for the Reverend Schulze, and even presented the case in a meeting of the Society.

According to this series of letters, members of the Society even tried to convince Dr. Ullman, the psychiatrist who was the Prince George's County psychiatrist who examined Ronald the second time, to talk about the case in the Society's meeting, but he refused due to the confidentiality of the case for the hospital. They also talked to Dr. Mabel Ross, who examined Ronald the first time, and tried to convince her to talk about the case. According to a letter dated July 5, 1949, she expressed great interest in the case and seemed willing to be convinced that there was something unusual about Ronald.

However, the Society members were concerned about the local reputation of the clinic. In the same series of letters, it was noted, "However they do not wish to discuss the case without permission from the parties concerned."[14]

Interestingly, the Society held a meeting with about 200 participants to present Ronald Hunkeler's case. Dick Darnell mentions that when the case was discussed before a scientist by the name of Lincoln, "I saw Lincoln's mouth drop open a couple of times and for a while I think he was not at all certain that we were serious" (letter dated June 7, 1949).[15] Also, the Society wanted to let the case be known to the public via the media before the Jesuits would do it. Therefore, they presented a press release where they tied the name of J.B. Rhine to the case, in which he was quoted as having said that the Ronald Hunkeler case was the most impressive poltergeist case that had come to his attention (letter dated August 17, 1949)[16]

It is important to note that all the above information about Ronald Hunkeler, the possessed boy, came from an extensive correspondence between Dr. Rhine of Duke University's Parapsychology Laboratory, and the Reverend Schulze, whose home he visited at some point to personally investigate the case.

16

Conclusion

This is perhaps the most difficult part for me to write about since I have a great deal of information on the Mount Rainier Exorcism, a case so controversial with so many facets to explore. What can we determine about this case that can constitute a final conclusion about *The Exorcist* and the Mount Rainier Exorcism? How can we present the facts clearly for the reader to reach a personal conclusion about the case?

However, the main purpose of this book is to provide as much information as possible on the most famous case of demonic possession in history. Consequently, the reader can gain a better understanding of what really lies behind the actual case and reach his or her own conclusions regarding the authenticity of this case as well as the underlying religious and moral message that William Peter Blatty wanted to convey in his book.

Nevertheless, even more important for me is how to understand demonic possession and exorcism in the light of science. Secondly, how to address those issues that involve the moral and religious aspects, as well as how both the Mount Rainier case and *The Exorcist* can influence our belief systems regarding matters of faith. I have also tried to convey how we perceive good and evil as the eternal dilemma we humans have faced throughout history, in the context of a dramatized story.

Up to this point I have been very critical of the Mount Rainier case. In general, I believe it could be explained by several hypotheses other than the demonic agency hypothesis (which in turn, cannot be proved in an indisputable manner to be absent), such as those evaluated in this case. However, in this final section, I would like to ask: What was it that was in control of Ronald? There is a certain phenomenal experience witnessed by some of the participants that, taken as a whole, make it almost impossible that men of good faith such as the Reverend Schulze, Father William Bowdern, and Father Raymond Bishop could have been entirely deceived by the adolescent named Ronald.

As mentioned before, the spontaneous and numerous marks that appeared on the boy's body, and the dramatic movement of the bed, if the reports are truthful and the witnesses reliable, provide evidence of phenomena that can hardly be explained by science—that actually lie beyond it, and do not fit with what is known by the current laws of medicine and psychology or the so-called "limiting principles of science." However, as explained in the model proposed by John Nicola in his book *Diabolical Possession*, I will next determine the most viable explanations to account for the way that participants experienced the case.

1. The Fraud Hypothesis

One theory about poltergeist activity or phenomena, such as the one manifested in the Mount Rainier case, is that they are simply childish pranks. Proponents of this view point out that it explains why so many poltergeist cases center around an adolescent, surrounded by unusual movement of objects, and why it is so rare for people to witness the initial stages of the movements of a displaced object. However, in this particular case, it is my contention that the poltergeist hypothesis is neither completely fraudulent nor genuine, but that it is a mixture of both. Also, after evaluating the evidence, some phenomena appear to be genuine. However, the adolescent undoubtedly committed fraud; for instance, at one point, Ronald was caught trying to deceive the exorcists. This type of fraud applies particularly to the first part of the events, before the formal rite of exorcism performed by Father William Bowdern and Father Bishop.

Furthermore, I am almost certain that some of the marks that appeared "apparently spontaneously" on Ronald's body (some of which appeared in the initial stages of the ordeal) were fraudulent: He had a motive for producing the marks on his own body, since he did not want to attend school and wanted to go to visit his aunt in St. Louis. Moreover, most of the marks that appeared on his body took place while he was out of the sight of his family members and the priests. Interestingly, the initial marks were seen and evaluated by the Reverend Schulze and his medical doctor, and Schulze declared that he never saw any specific marks in the form of letters (as the family claimed), only nerve rashes. It is my opinion that the adolescent made some of the marks himself to avoid going to school. I think that fraud accounts for about 20 percent of the phenomena in the Mount Rainier Exorcism case.

2. The Natural Hypothesis (Especially Psychological)

For many experts in mental health and psychological disorders can explain cases of demonic possession. Bromwell declared (2008)[1]: "Belief in the possibility of demonic possession has waned since the advent of sophisticated medical knowledge. What had previously been considered to be examples of control of an individual by a spirit or devil are now commonly accepted as numerous forms of mental illness, easily explained by nervous system activity" (p. 1).

Regarding the hypothesis above, I believe the conversion disorder diagnosis to be valid along with some malingering on the part of the adolescent in this case. Also, Tourette's disorder and its main syndrome coprolalia (the uncontrolled and unfettered utterance of profanities) may account for the adolescent's screaming of obscene and foul language. Moreover, from the very beginning of the ordeal, the first medical evaluation that took place found the following diagnosis: Dr. Mabel Rose of the University of Maryland's mental health clinic indicated that "the boy did not to want to grow up and assume responsibility, but preferred holding onto his childhood" (letter from the Reverend Schulze to J.B. Rhine, dated September 19, 1949).[2] Ronald had two medical evaluations at the psychiatric unit at the University of Maryland, and a third one scheduled as a follow-up, which he missed. I am certain that the psychiatrist who evaluated Ronald may have carried out a clinical evaluation and, based on the symptoms, rendered his medical diagnosis.

The key conclusion here is "that the boy did not want to … assume responsibility." This is congruent with the diagnosis of conversion disorder, in which the individual tries to avoid unpleasant stimuli or responsibility, in this case attending school, which is a sign of maturity. Had the doctors conducted a battery of psychological personality tests and complementary clinical studies, they would very likely have confirmed the conversion disorder diagnosis. Interestingly, at this stage of the case, the Reverend Schulze and his personal physician examined the initial markings—the letters that appeared on the boy's body. However, in his letter to J.B. Rhine on March 21, 1949, Schulze indicated that they did not see letters, but instead saw marks that seemed like nerve rashes.[3] This is the key in determining (in the initial evaluation) that it is unlikely that any clear words ever appeared on the boy's body, at least at this time in the case. In my personal opinion, the psychological hypothesis accounts for approximately 35 percent of the phenomena manifested in this case.

3. The Poltergeist Hypothesis

Many experts believe that demonic possession cases are actually poltergeist phenomena with demonic persecution as a complementary element. A few cases are even of vicious character with sustained persecution of a particular individual or family. These cases often have a religious element, and they may focus on a clergyman and feature desecration of religious objects. This is the main difference with poltergeist cases. In the Mount Rainier Exorcism, I believe the case presents the features of a conventional poltergeist case, and that it became a possession case after the decision to perform the exorcism. It is important to note that after the fraud hypothesis, the second line of investigation of the case was that it could be a poltergeist-like phenomenon. In spite of the fact that he was not a parapsychologist, the Rev. Luther Schulze was familiar with the work of J.B. Rhine, who asked for a report of the case. Rhine then contacted Dick Darnell, president of the Society for Parapsychology, who in turn recommended that Schulze proceed with an investigation. Darnell offered Schulze a stenographer to assist with writing initial reports on the case for Rhine.

The aforementioned reports were prepared by his church administrative assistant Ida Mae Donley. Also, Darnell organized a meeting of the Society to present the case as a "conventional poltergeist case." It is important to note, however, that the poltergeist hypothesis is difficult to exclude as a causal etiology of some of the phenomena surrounding the Mount Rainier Exorcism. The phenomena witnessed by the Rev. Luther Schulze, particularly the movement of the bed and a heavy armchair, strongly suggest that paranormal activity may have taken place. Moreover, in a letter to J.B. Rhine dated March 21, 1949, Schulze described that "his bed shook whenever the adolescent was on it with him. As he described it, when he was in the bed with me mine vibrated ... there was no apparent motion of his body."[4] Also, in the report sent to Rhine, the psychokinetic effect reported by Schulze was much more dramatic: "When the adolescent spent the night at his premises, once in bed ... Schulze heard the boy's bed creaking. He noticed Ronald was still awake.... He put his hand and felt Ronald's bed shaking like one of those motel vibrator beds, but much faster. The boy was still, his limbs and head and body were perfectly still but the bed was shaking."[5]

Also, when Father Bishop, one of the exorcists, visited Ronald, as reported by Thomas Allen in *Possessed* (1993),[6] "He saw Robbie's [Ronald's] mattress moving back and forth ... the boy lay perfectly still ... and did not exert any physical efforts. The movement in one direction did not exceed more than three inches, the action was intermittent and completed subsided after a period of approximately 15 minutes" (p. 55).

The aforementioned descriptions of the dramatic movement of the mattress, by skeptical minister the Reverend Schulze and by Father Bishop, may constitute a "smoking gun" or evidence suggesting it is very likely that poltergeist-like phenomena may have really taken place. When I interviewed the Reverend Schulze in 1990, he expressed that he did not consider this to be a demonic possession case nor a poltergeist case even though he knew the work of J.B. Rhine at Duke University on parapsychology. All he would admit was that there was some kind of phenomena that for him was very hard to explain via scientific means. I also consider that the poltergeist phenomena constitute a better explanatory hypothesis than a demonic possession hypothesis, if the phenomena of moving of objects as witnessed by Father Bowdern and the Reverend Schulze are truthful and really took place. I would give 40 percent probability to the poltergeist hypothesis in explaining, as a model, the physical phenomena surrounding the case such as the movement of objects, including beds and the like.

4. The Demonic Possession Hypothesis

The Vatican guidelines stress that most behaviors that appear to be caused by demonic possession are actually triggered by psychiatric illness. Monsignor Corrado Balducci, the Vatican's former chief exorcist, estimated that only 5 or 6 out of every thousand people who seek help from an exorcist are really possessed by evil spirits. The remainder are in need of psychiatric help.[7]

Does the Mount Rainier case fall within these 5 or 6 out of 1,000 cases? I would say it's unlikely. However, let us analyze this hypothesis. First, as I indicated before, the devil would have to exist as an independent entity "as the Catholic Church has defined his existence" in order to accept demonic possession as such. However, the existence of the devil cannot be proved indisputably. If you believe in the Catholic doctrine of the existence of the devil and exorcism as the cure for cases of demonic possession, then this would be a classic case of demonic possession. Nevertheless, its existence has not been proved and your belief would constitute a matter of faith. As indicated by Warwick (1976)[8]: "The reality of exorcism thus depends squarely on the reality of (1) demons and (2) demon possession. If there is no personal supernatural evil, then clearly there are no demons to possess people and no genuine exorcism of demons. Moreover, if the Devil exists, if they did not enter and control humans' personalities, exorcism would be purposeless" (pp. 1183–1185).

Moreover, looking carefully at the case, we will find that the Mount Rainier Exorcism was considered to be, possibly, a conventional poltergeist case when it was still in the hands of the Rev. Luther Schulze. However, once the exorcism was introduced, possession began. The devil was not present on the scene of the case until after they decided to perform an exorcism; in other words, when it fell in the hands of the Catholic priests. For the Reverend Schulze, however, this was only a case with some "extraordinary strange phenomena" that he could not explain and this is why he consulted J.B. Rhine in order to find a possible answer. Perhaps if they had not decided that the case was "extraordinary" and the Jesuits had not rendered a case or possession, *The Exorcist* would have had never existed, either as a book or a movie.

Furthermore, in order to be considered a case of demonic possession, as far as the Catholic Church outlines it in the Roman Ritual, the same priests went ahead with the exorcism when it was clear to them that it was a case of obsession, just as a preventive measure before the case reached the possession stage. If this was the case, instead of helping Ronald, they made a terrible mistake and it is likely that these actions led the boy to believe that he was possessed, so he acted accordingly. Suggestion is a powerful tool. In his book *El rostro oculto de la mente* (*The Hidden Face of Mind*), the Jesuit Oscar Gonzalez Quevedo relates a case in which, during an experiment of suggestibility, a woman is told that she is losing a lot of blood; after being pinched on one of her arms, which was out of her sight, almost immediately she suffered a heart attack.[9] Thus, I would not be surprised that if Ronald was told that he was possessed by a demon, he would act accordingly. In other words, the Catholic priests injected the idea of the demon into his mind with the rituals of exorcism. I am almost certain that the demonic hypothesis does not hold in this case. I would grant a 5 percent possibility of this hypothesis to have actually taken place and 100 percent to conclude that they converted this case of apparent poltergeist phenomena into one of demonic possession. I would exclude this hypothesis to be on the top of the hierarchy of explanations to investigate demonic possession cases as suggested by Father John Nicola in his book *Diabolical Possession and Exorcism*. Although I am not a dogmatic writer, based on the analysis of the case, I find the likelihood of demonic possession as a causal explanation is very low. However, the possibility is always there of a demonic agency hypothesis to be valid, since no one can prove that this was totally impossible in the Mount Rainier case. Nevertheless, the demonic agency hypothesis is very improbable, although not impossible.

Finally, I would say that the Mount Rainier case is permeated to some extent with a mixture of all of the above hypotheses, some more likely to explain the real causes of the phenomena in question than others. To conclude, Nicola's theoretical model, presented in *Diabolical Possession and Exorcism*, put forth to better evaluate cases of demonic possession, has been applied here in the context of the Mount Rainier case. The four explanations or hypotheses of the hierarchy of causality proposed by Nicola provide us with a broader perspective to better understand the phenomena of diabolical possession and exorcism than any other approaches that I have evaluated so far. Consequently, following Nicola to evaluate cases of demonic possession, if we can exclude the first three possibilities (fraud, parapsychological phenomena, natural or psychological phenomena), then the fourth possibility appears as the most likely explanation, so we will then consider the demonic agency hypothesis as the causal factor. In this particular case, however, I believe we cannot indisputably exclude the first three hypotheses. Therefore, this case can most likely be explained in the context of the Principle of Scientific Economy, which can paraphrased: when a natural and ordinary explanation is possible, we do not have to resort to unusual and extraordinary causes even though the potentiality, and the possibility, are always there (Nicola, 1974).[10]

In other words, there are plenty of indicators in the case that natural explanations such as fraud (either intentionally or unconsciously) may have been part of the Mount Rainier case. Also, the case nicely fits the conversion reaction diagnosis, as applied to Ronald, in which a person can obtain benefits from a psychological condition. It is also difficult to exclude the parapsychological hypothesis as a causal etiology of some of the phenomena. If we could include poltergeist as a natural or ordinary explanation as part of the entire model to explain the phenomena along with the fraud and psychological hypothesis, then we would have a 95 percent validity of the actual causes of the phenomena surrounding the Mount Rainier exorcism via natural scientific explanations.

However, poltergeist-like phenomena have been rejected by scientists who believe in the so-called "limiting principles of science," by which these phenomena do not fit the current laws of science that we accept at the present time. Yet the same issue occurred when we accepted Newtonian physics as absolute laws of the universe; any theories that did not fit this paradigm were denied by the scientific community. However, with the discovery of the theory of relativity by Einstein, our vision of the world has changed, and may open us up to the possibility that these types of anomalistic phenomena may actually take place.

We cannot completely prove nor deny that the Mount Rainier case was an incidence of demonic possession. Although the evidence in this case for such an occurrence to have taken place is very slim and weak, such a possibility cannot be denied. As stated in the "Hamlet principle of science": "All is possible in the universe."

I will complete this conclusion with two comments, one from the realm of religion and the other one from science. First, regarding the belief in the existence of the devil and demonic possession, Cardinal Jorge Medina Estevez stressed: "However, the Church is not going soft on the belief of Satan and his demons … the existence of the devil isn't an opinion, something to take or leave as you wish. Anyone who says he doesn't exist would not have the fullness of the Catholic faith … the devil's presence is seen in the widespread acceptance of lies and deceit. The idolatry of money.… The idolatry of sex … the presence of the devil … explains the dramatic condition of the world, which languishes under the power of the malign one" (2010, Ontario Consultants).[11]

Regarding the above reference, that the devil is reflected in our own humanity and deeds, when I asked a friend of mine, a pastor of my church, if he believed in the devil, he replied to me, "In my opinion the worst devils are humans. I think the 'other' is the Devil." I think that this latter part of what Cardinal Estevez asserts constitutes the spinal cord of the doctrine of the existence of the devil. The human condition becomes malignant under the influence of the devil, which has deteriorated the values of society with wars, exploitation of the disadvantaged, and injustices of many kinds. It seems to me that this message is more important than whether or not the devil or demonic possession exists, which is, of course, a matter of faith for those who believe it.

This is the message that William Peter Blatty wanted to convey in his dramatization of the real story in order to cause social change. Blatty was certain that he did not have all the information and that it was likely that the story he used was not totally true. However, it served him as a springboard for providing a memorable moral message about the values of a deteriorated American society in the early 1970s.

Regarding the scientific or religious aspect, no one will ever be able to demonstrate solely from this case that demonic possession does or does not exist. As I indicated previously, this is more a matter of faith. Nevertheless, experts coming from a scientific background, such as Melissa A. Bromwell, have been open to the possibility that the phenomenon of demonic possession may be a viable explanation not yet understood by science. As she expressed regarding the phenomena surrounding cases of demonic possession:

> However, there is quite a bit about supposed demonic possession which cannot yet be explained by biology. This category includes such phenomena as levitation, wounds appearing upon the victim that have not been inflicted by the self or another concrete source, knowledge of languages never before studied, sometimes never even heard, and psychic abilities such as knowing facts about other individuals that have never been met. In addition, the accompanying situations related to the area around possessed individuals do not seem to be explainable in terms of the brain or any aspect of biology; science cannot yet explain the distinct decrease in temperature of the room the individual occupies, the appearance of writing and sounds from an unseen force, and the movement of objects on their own (Bromwell, 2008, p. 1).

Also, according to Bromwell, we can come to two conclusions regarding demonic possession: First, that someday, "science via further studies by brain science may explain the phenomena surrounding a supposed possessed person. If so, then this may reveal that there is something biologically (and entirely secular) unique about such individuals which allows them to be capable of creating such phenomena by themselves; in this case it could be determined that demonic possession is nothing but a myth perpetuated for centuries."

Second, on the other hand, she believed that "the possibility that demonic possession is a real occurrence cannot yet be rejected; no thoroughly decisive evidence exists to the contrary. What is currently known about science cannot fully explain every situation reported to be a case of demonic possession, at least not by the methods which science currently employs. Until science can explain each detail, if indeed it ever can, one cannot dismiss the possibility that demonic possession is a real and true phenomenon" (p. 1).[12]

In other words, even though there is currently an accepted principle of science which states that we do not have to rely on a supernatural explanation if we have a natural one, on the other hand, the Hamlet principle proposes that all is possible. Until then, dogmatic "scientific positions" so far expressed by many writers on *The Exorcist* as well as the Mount Rainier Exorcism would contribute better to human knowledge with a critical mind rather than a dogmatic mind.

Appendix A

The Letters Between the
Rev. Luther Miles Schulze
and Dr. J.B. Rhine

In this addendum, I include the transcribed information from the original letters of the correspondence between the Rev. Luther Miles Schulze and the director of Duke's Parapsychology Laboratory, psychologist Dr. J.B. Rhine. I will make some personal comments at the bottom of each letter.

Letter A

St. Stephen's Evangelical Lutheran Church

March 21, 1949

Dear Dr. Rhine:

We have in our congregation a family who are being disturbed by Poltergeist phenomena. It first appeared about January 15, 1949. The family consists of the maternal grandmother, a fourteen year old boy who is an only child, and his parents. The phenomena are apparent only in the boy's presence. I had him in my home on the night of February 17–18 to observe for myself. Chairs moved with him and one threw him out. His bed shook whenever he was in it. When he was in bed with me, mine vibrated. There was no apparent motion of his body. I then made a bed on the floor for him and this glided over the floor.

The family lives in Prince George's County, Maryland, so I had their physician place the boy in the hands of the County Mental Hygiene Clinic, under Dr. Mabel Ross of the University of Maryland. She and her staff had two interviews with the boy. He was to have gone for a third, but meantime words appeared on the boy's body, according to the family and friends. My physician and I saw no words, but we did see nerve reaction rashes which had the appearance of scratches. The words indicated to the family that they should take the boy to St. Louis. They were originally from there. They said the words wrote in him that they should go for three and a half weeks!! Now he has visions of the devil and goes into a trance and speaks in a strange language, they tell me.

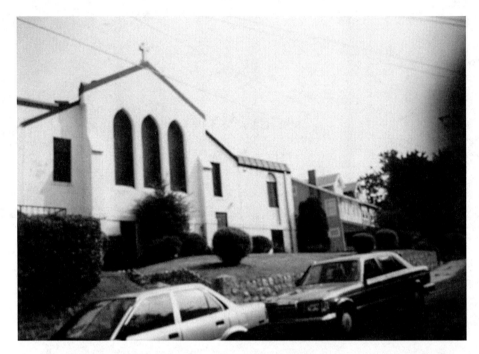

St. Stephen's Evangelical Lutheran Church (in 1993), ministered by the Reverend Luther Miles Schulze back in 1949. This is the church that Ronald attended with his family, and where the circle of prayers was organized by Ida Mae Donley on his behalf. Located at 1611 Brentwood Road, N.E., Washington, D.C.

I am insisting that the family return here to their home and put the boy into a hospital under the care of a physician who is sympathetic to the case. My physician is sympathetic. Theirs went to the mental hygiene clinic only after insistence and persisted in trying to treat the boy with Barbital.

Would you, or someone from your staff, be interested in studying this case here after the family returns? If not, can you recommend some competent person who will do it? Would you want someone from Harvard University, too, or do you prefer to investigate alone?

The family mentioned other such phenomena as chairs moving, tables over-turning, objects flying through the air, and scratching and drummings. Their floors are scarred from sliding of heavy furniture.

I case you wish to contact the family at their temporary address:

Mr. and Mrs. Edwin C. Hunkeler
c/o L.C. Hunkeler
8435 Roanoke Drive,
Normandy, Missouri

Very truly yours
Luther Miles Schulze

Comments

The Reverend Schulze, who was skeptical about what had been reported to him by the family, reports "surprising phenomena" that take place right in front of him. Interestingly, the reporting of a bed vibrating, when he was on it with the boy, represents a very surprising phenomenon hard to explain by any current scientific law. He also reports that "there was no apparent motion of the adolescent's body" such as would cause such a phenomenon. He also explains that the marks that indicated that the boy had to be taken to St. Louis were not actual letter marks, but that they looked more like nerve rashes that had the appearance of scratches. This last observation by the Reverend Schulze likely indicates that these marks may have been self-inflicted by the adolescent or perhaps caused by a stress reaction. A medication for epileptic seizures is also prescribed at this stage of the case.

Letter B

March 23, 1949

Dear Mr. Schulze:

Your most interesting letter has come in the absence of my husband, who will be out of the city until the end of this week. I hasten to reply, however, because I am certain that he will be intensely interested in the case you mention. I am sure that he will want to study the case, if possible, at the earliest opportunity. I also believe that at the start he would prefer to be alone and also to avoid newspaper publicity. Doubtless you and the family also will concur in that.

I hope you will be able to persuade the family to return to their home. It would surely seem that your idea of having the boy under the care of a sympathetic physician is best one. Unfortunately, there are probably very few who would really understand a case like this, and if you know of one who would, they would be fortunate, indeed, to have the boy under his care.

For the present I suppose it is not necessary that I contact the family personally; but I hope that you will express to them our strong interest, both in the unusual case and in the welfare of the child. If there is anything more that could be done to reassure them of our understanding and the competence to come in on the case, I hope you will do it. Please keep us informed of anything new that comes to your attention, and I will report to Mr. Rhine as soon as he returns.

Sincerely yours,
(Mrs. J.B. Rhine)

Comments

Dr. Louisa Rhine, the wife of J.B. Rhine, responds to the letter in the absence of her husband. She was a co-researcher at the Institute for Parapsychology and personally investigated the case by visiting the premises of Dr. Reverend Schulze in Washington, D.C.

Letter C

April 2, 1949

Dear Mr. Schulze:

I am writing you briefly just to support what Mrs. Rhine wrote you. I am deeply interested in this case and want to help in any way I can. I think Dr. Winfred Overholzer at St. Elizabeth might take an interest in the case, but it might be best to wait until the family returns and you can see whether any changes in the situation have occurred. Sometimes these phenomena stop abruptly.

I will be going through Washington several times this spring and could stop off if I know it would be of any help.

As you know, the most likely normal explanation is that the boy is, himself, led to create the effect of being the victim of mysterious agencies or forces and might be sincerely convinced of it. Such movements as those of the chair and the bed might, from your very brief account of them, have originated within himself. Presumably, however, the movement of the bed in the floor was not of that type. I presume you observed the movement in good light and were not in any way relying upon his account of it.

I am sufficiently interested that if you find those phenomena occurring in your presence and are yourself convinced of their parapsychological character, I would like to go right up to join you in making whatever study of them is possible and doing whatever we can to relieve the boy. I wish you would telephone me with reverse charges if, when the boy returns, there is still a recurrence of the type of phenomena we are discussing, and especially if you can get him for a time under your control or that of your physician.

Sincerely yours,

J.B. Rhine

Comments

This is a most interesting letter, in which Dr. J.B. Rhine lays out the hypothesis that the adolescent may be under suggestion and, therefore, convinced that he was "the victim of mysterious agencies or forces." Also, he cannot explain the nature of the movement of the bed made on the floor and observed by the Reverend. He shows his interest in investigating this case personally, a trip that he actually made to the premises of the Reverend Schulze in Washington, D.C., where these phenomena took place.

Letter D

April 6, 1949

Dear Dr. Rhine:

Thank you for your letter of April 2. Please address further mail as indicated because it saves a little time.

The Hunkeler family has returned from St. Louis. While out there, at various times, an Episcopal priest and Lutheran pastor were approached on this matter. The

Jesuits were also contacted and they admitted that it was the devil and finally had a service of exorcism. The boy appears perfectly healthy despite the three months of antics with loss of sleep. The Jesuit here wants to place him in the monastery and hold services for 21 days.

I have given them the names of two very devout Christian women, one of whom holds prayer circles regularly in her home in which some illnesses have been cured. The other is the daughter in law of Dr. Vincent, Presbyterian missionary to China, who had experiences with similar cases.

Frankly, I do not know what the family wishes to do. They have only been home about thirty hours. They are a bit skeptical about anyone from a university, especially a psychiatrist! They feel this is entirely a religious problem. Unfortunately, while they were in St. Louis a relative attending Washington University brought someone from the faculty to the house, who told them of his fantasies concerning the spirit world; that someday we could tune in any of the departed we wished to, just as we now tune in a television program.

I wish that I could give you some definite plan now. Perhaps I can later. Thank you and best wishes.

Sincerely yours,
Luther M. Schulze

Comments

Clearly, in this letter the Jesuits "had diagnosed the case as one of demonic possession and carried out the exorcism." Also, this letter proves the suggestibility attitude of the family, reluctant to accept the help of a professional psychiatrist to solve the problem. The Reverend Schulze laments that a friend of the family from a university, who visited them, even strengthened the family's superstitious beliefs.

Letter E

St. Stephen's Evangelical Lutheran Church

April 19, 1949

Dear Dr. Rhine:

Thank you for trying to contact me today, but I thought if you could save the expense of this call by writing to you since I was out for several hours anyway.

Mrs. Hunkeler and her son returned to St. Louis on April 8. Two Jesuits had come here with them, tried to place the boy in a hospital, claimed they could find no place and influenced her to return to St. Louis with them. The Jesuits say they will place the boy in one of their hospitals there. The family appears to have great confidence in the Latin Ritual and the tales of experience in exorcism told them by the priest.

I have a feeling that the family needs treatment as individuals and as a family eventually and that we will be expected to pick up the pieces. If you come to Washington in the near future I will be happy to talk a few hours at your convenience and give you more details even though there seem to be nothing we can do at the present ... boy sleeping in rectory in last report.

Thank you again. Best Wishes
Sincerely yours
Luther Miles Schulze

Comments

At this point in the case, the family had accepted the ritual of exorcism and the adolescent was placed in the Alexian Brothers Hospital in St. Louis, Missouri, where the final exorcism took place.

Letter F

April 21, 1949

Dear Mr. Schulze:

I have put in a telephone call for you for this afternoon, but it may turn out that I will not get to talk with you, and here is a bit of the written word to make sure we keep in close touch on this delicate matter.

Could you give me an account of the firsthand evidence you have of these phenomena—what you actually saw the boy do or witnessed in his presence? If I could be entirely sure that the phenomena are not explainable by trickery, conscious or unconscious, I would try to work my way into direct contact, and I think it would be possible through one means or another. Your help would, of course, be very important. The reason I take this guarded position is that a number of these cases have been reduced to clever trickery, and since we are not ordinarily prepared for the unusual sort (rather, pathological) of faking that is sometimes practiced, we are not as guarded as would be required to see everything that is going on.

What I have put in the telephone call to clear up is just this matter of how good the evidence is—that something really difficult to explain is going go.

It is too bad to have the inter-denominational confusion introduced that you refer to. It suggests that we are still in the Middle Ages, as, indeed, many of us are.

I am going to be gone from Duke from the twenty-second (3 p.m.) to the evening of the fourth. I will, however, be in Baltimore on the third but will have to make good time driving from Baltimore to Durham, as I have to arrive by the evening of the fourth. In case anything comes up that I need to be reached at Baltimore, I will be at the Stafford Hotel. I am lecturing for the Society of Hygiene at 8 p.m. on the third. If you need any help in this investigation from people there is Washington who are interested, you might want to make contact with Mr. Richard Darnell, President of the Society for Parapsychology, who is at 915 Eighteenth Street, N.W.

His home telephone is Axminister 7039. I do not know his office telephone number.

Sincerely Yours
J.B. Rhine

Comments

This is a very clever letter. In this one Dr. J.B. Rhine outlines the approach to be followed on the investigation of this type of case in order to prove that the phenomena of ostensible paranormal phenomena reported, is not a hoax or fraud. He suggests to the Reverend Schulze that he conduct a careful assessment of the case to make sure that the phenomena are genuine and not the result of trickery, either conscious or unconscious. The unconscious trickery, if this was the case, suits the conversion reaction diagnosis of the case, as we presented it in the natural explanation hypothesis of the case.

Letter G

April 21, 1949

Dear Mr. Schulze:

Thank you for your note, which reached me before I left. With my present plans in mind it seems unlikely that I will be able to stop in Washington for more than a brief chat, possibly only a telephone call, unless I am able to get a good start from Baltimore. If I do not I may not come through Washington, awaiting a day visit.

So far I have not been able to think of anyone in St. Louis who could take charge. I hope you will collect all the information you can about this curious case and the curious treatment being applied. Few people would believe that either one could occur.

Sincerely yours,
J.B. Rhine

Letter H

July 1, 1949

Dear Pastor Schulze:

We are very much indebted to you for the trouble to which you have gone in preparing the report of the of the Ronald case. Dick Darnell has just sent me a copy.

It seems to me that you did everything that an intelligent, capable minister could have done under the circumstances, and I am greatly impressed by the real service you gave the family. This is true ministry.

There were a few details in your oral account that I do not find in your written report. I may, of course, have been mistaken or you may have forgotten these when you dictated the story:

First paragraph on pg. 4 of the report: Was the light on in the room? The paragraph preceding is not entirely clear in this point. [Schulze handwrote his answers to the first questions in black ink on the typewritten letter: Answer: Yes]

A second question I should like to know about is where you were located while the chair was overturned. [standing in front when it toppled]

I take it you made no attempt to catch the boy as he fell over. I wonder why if you recall? Would you mind telling me what your emotion were if you can remember? [I wanted to see if it would really go over.]

Dick tells me that you have the Jesuits' report. That should be interesting.

Now have a more serious question. It is raised by two considerations. The first is that this story is gradually going to reach out everywhere, and if so, it is a good plan to have at least a brief statement of the essential facts in some form that can be made available to serious students and inquirers. The other circumstance is that Dick tells me you have consented to talk to the Society about the case next fall. This leads me to suggest that an outline of the story be presented in the Parapsychology Bulletin, with all proper consideration for protection of the parties concerned. It seems to me that this could be worked out so that there would be no embarrassment to anyone. It would on other hand, furnish a convenient way of informing the people who most ought to know about the Ronald case. Whether or not your name would appear would be for you to decide.

You could come to a decision after the condensation is prepared and the general tone and effect and can be appraised. For my part, I think it would not detract from the report to have your name withheld, but on the other hand, I do not think it would hurt your work or the family for your name to be used. Of course the family name would not be given.

At any rate, I would like to know what you think about this; and since I am sending a copy to Dick for his reaction, we will know what he thinks also. Whether the statement is published in our July number or three months later is immaterial, though I think the sooner the better from the point of view of cutting in on any rumor or lurid tales that may break out in the Sunday supplements.

I have a constructive interest in publication. I would like everyone who studies our literature to be alert to the importance of such cases and to the need of informing us at the earliest possible point of any case encountered. One such seed might someday bring us a bushel of fruit. I think of the way in which such a case is handle by different churches.

Sincerely yours,
J.B. Rhine

Comments

Dr. J.B. Rhine was interested in making the case public via the Washington Society for Parapsychology so that people would know how these cases are handled by the different churches. However, before doing so, he questions the Reverend Schulze regarding the measures he had taken when he witnessed the phenomena, seeking for certainty of the events before proceeding to publish it in in the *Parapsychology Bulletin*. He wanted to make sure the Reverend Schulze, a man of good faith, had not been deceived by trickery and to ascertain the authenticity of the phenomena related by the Reverend to him. Once the case was reported by the Parapsychology Society of Washington, it was also reported by the *Washington Post*. William Blatty became aware of the case via the *Washington Post*, from which he reimagined it to create the novel *The Exorcist*.

Letter I

St. Stephen's Evangelical Lutheran Church
September 19, 1949

Dear Dr. Rhine:

Your letter dated the 15th and postmarked the 17th reached me this morning. However, because of a busy schedule, it is doubtful if I could have accepted your gracious invitation to come to Durham this week or any time in the very near future.

About the release to the press, I had some misgivings at the time it was discussed about doing so. Mr. Darnell's purpose was to inform people of the existence of the Parapsychology Society so that if and when unusual phenomena appeared witnesses would contact the society.

In the case that I reported it may interest to you to know that I saw the boy in June. He had grown taller, gained weight, his neck has thickened and his voice deepened. I have an idea that medical examinations would show that he reached puberty during his experience. The family is still living in fear of recurrence and was quite distressed at the newspaper publicity even though their identity was concealed.

The report from the mental hygiene clinic, where the family took the boy for two appointments but failed to follow through on the third, indicates that the boy did seem to want go grow up and assume responsibility, but preferred holding on to his childhood.

I know nothing about the Petersburg case. Someone, I cannot recall who, told me that Johns Hopkins Hospital had issued a statement that a heretofore un-named physical ailment produced body antics similar to those mentioned by Catholic priests in cases of "demoniacs."

Thank you again. Best wishes and kindest regards.

Sincerely yours,
Luther Miles Schulze

Comments

A fascinating report of the mental status of the adolescent, before the case was diagnosed as one of demonic possession, had been presented by medical doctors of the mental health hygiene clinic in Maryland. From this report, we can infer that he did not want to assume responsibility but preferred to hold onto his childhood. In other words, this supports the hypothesis that he suffered from conversion reaction, whereby the person suffers from psychosomatic mental and physical illnesses to avoid confronting what they consider a negative stimulus. In the case of Ronald, he did not want to go to school.

Letter J

September 21, 1949

Dear Dr. Schulze,

The puberty hypothesis is the one to watch in these cases. If you can get anything further from the Johns Hopkins rumor, I wish you would pass it on to me. There is a twelve-year-old boy in the Petersburg family I mentioned.

Thank you again. Best wishes and kindest regards

Sincerely yours,
J.B. Rhine

Appendix B

Interview with the Rev. Luther Miles Schulze and Ruth Schulze

Introduction

One night on June 22, 1990, I decided to call a retirement home belonging to the Lutheran Church, located in Rockville, Maryland. I had just received the grant to research the case on which William Peter Blatty had based his celebrated novel and subsequent film *The Exorcist*. As part of my research investigation, I was also interested in finding out if the people involved in the actual case were still alive and whether I would be allowed to interview them. I realized that it was going to be hard to find witnesses who were still alive, since it had been 40 years since the original incident took place. However, I also thought I had nothing to lose by trying to find them. At the suggestion of Anne Carrol, business manager at the Foundation for Research on the Nature of Man, who assisted me in this investigation, I decided to call the Lutheran Synod in Maryland. To my surprise, I found that one of the main witnesses of the Mount Rainier case, the Rev. Luther Miles Schulze, was still alive and living at their retirement home.

When I called the admissions office of the retirement home, the person in charge confirmed that the Reverend Schulze was one of their residents, along with his wife Ruth, and that my call could be transferred his room despite its being late, around 9 p.m. Honestly, it had never occurred to me that one of the main witnesses would still be alive. I had read the fascinating letters of the Reverend Schulze to Dr. J.B. Rhine, written back in 1949. When they transferred my call to his room, I was quite nervous and excited, never imagining that the Rev. Luther Schulze himself would answer the call. This conversation with the Reverend Schulze that night was the beginning of one of the most fascinating adventures in my life, experiencing a piece of the living history of the actual Mount Rainier Exorcism, the event that Blatty's novel was based on.

However, it is important to note that the Reverend Schulze was the initial

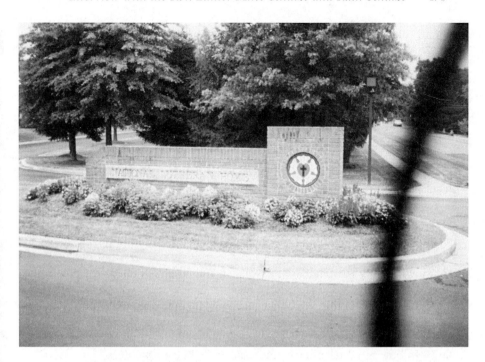

Entrance (in 1993) of the National Lutheran Home located in Rockville, Maryland, the place where I interviewed the Reverend Schulze and his wife and became acquainted with members of the circle of prayers that were organized on behalf of Ronald Hunkeler.

trained cleric to be contacted and entrusted with the case by the family of the reportedly possessed adolescent. Schulze was an honest man with a scientifically oriented perspective and conducted a very objective investigation of the initial phenomena surrounding the Mount Rainier case. He decided to call in the most famous and prestigious researcher of the paranormal at the time, Dr. J.B. Rhine, the father of modern scientific parapsychology, who at the time was the director of the parapsychology studies program at Duke University.

Moreover, he contacted his own physician to carry out a physical medical evaluation on the adolescent. In addition, he even recommended that the adolescent, by the name of "Ronald," be taken to a medical facility to complete a medical check-up of his physical and mental condition. Schulze did not right away believe as factual what the family told him about the strange paranormal phenomena surrounding the adolescent. Instead, he decided to find out on his own if the phenomena, of a "poltergeist" nature, were real and that the family was not being deceived or impressed by any type of suggestibility. In order to investigate this question, he asked the family that the adolescent stay at his premises one night to confirm if such phenomena really were occurring to the 14-year-old adolescent.

The Reverend Schulze was skeptical about the reported phenomena, and that night, he expected that "nothing would happen" in his apartment. To his surprise, he was shocked by the events that he would later witness, elements described in the interview that I conducted with him at the retirement home. Despite the dramatic paranormal events that he witnessed on that night, he took a gradual a skeptical approach and did not rush to judgment, eschewing a "demonic possession" hypothesis.

He realized that he needed to have a specialist on the phenomena to investigate the case, and therefore contacted Dr. J.B. Rhine, with whom he corresponded extensively on the case. He even invited Rhine and his wife, Dr. Louisa Rhine, to investigate the case at the premises. He held the belief that perhaps science could explain the phenomena surrounding the 14-year-old adolescent before turning to a supernatural agency hypothesis to explain it. However, his skeptical and scientific attitude was not liked very much by the family of the adolescent, who became disappointed with him, since he hesitated to believe the events that the family members related to him. Therefore, they decided to have him removed from the case, and instead presented their case to the Catholic Church.

In our initial telephone conversation, Schulze, who answered my call, asked my name and the reason why I was calling. I replied that I was a visiting scholar at the Foundation for Research on the Nature of Man, the former Duke parapsychology laboratory. I told him I was interested in a case that he may recall, which the movie *The Exorcist* was based on. He replied, "How could I forget?" Schulze remembered Dr. Rhine, a friend who even visited his home in the late 1950s. It was late and he had to sleep, never having talked to anyone about the case, even though he had been approached several times by reporters. He lauded my efforts and the foundation and ended by telling me, "I'll be glad to talk to you about the case."

The next day, I took a bus to the National Lutheran Home. The bus did not drop me off near the retirement home, and I had to take a rather long walk to get there. Once I arrived, I was asked to wait while they informed Schulze of my arrival. Shortly, I was asked to enter a special area for visitors and a room where the Reverend Schulze was waiting for me; he was in a wheelchair and looked physically fit. He greeted me by saying, "Look at this young man! He wants to take me to the past, a past that I do not want to recall or talk about again. But he seems like a good young man and he comes from a serious place, the Institute for Parapsychology. I have fond memories of his Director Dr. J.B. Rhine, a good friend of mine back in the late 1950s."

After he greeted me, he asked me to sit down and then inquired if my visit pertained to the Mount Rainier case. Upon finding about his involvement in the famous case, a couple of nurses and doctors who were present were really surprised, asking Schulze: "How come you never told us about it?" Another nurse jokingly replied, "I understand now why I felt strange when walking by your room." All of us laughed!

I then turned on my tape recorder and began the interview with Schulze in the presence of the medical doctor and a couple of nurses. As I was about to ask him the first question, he interrupted me and commented that there were some volunteers at the retirement home who had attended the church where he was a pastor in the 1950s, individuals who knew about the case in question. They had served as the members of the group who conducted the "circles of prayer" for the sake of Ronald's spiritual liberation. At that moment, an elderly woman arrived, Schulze's wife, informing us that she too remembered many of the details surrounding the case. This was a great added and unexpected help.

In addition, she divulged that Schulze had kept many of the details of the case in secrecy and had sent information only to the synod of the church. Then she confirmed that many of the volunteers who were also involved in the case would be available for interviewing. "Well," she told me, "once you talk to my husband then you can go down to the area where they are now and talk to them. Ida, one of the volunteers of our church and friends with the Hunkeler family, know where the family lived … and where the events took place." It is important to note that what impressed me the most about Schulze and his wife was the extraordinary memory they showed during this interview, even though so many years, almost a half century, had passed since the Mount Rainier Exorcism had taken place. This interview was recorded and notes were taken for complementary information not recorded on tape.

Interview with the Rev. Luther Miles Schulze at the National Lutheran Home: July 25, 1990

> Note: To facilitate a better understanding of some of the questions related to the case, I will provide an explanation in brackets to clarify what events in the case I am referring to when asking the questions. Also, I will further explain the events using excerpts from the actual letters sent to J.B. Rhine, information that will provide additional insights and complement the interview.

Background Information on the Case

In one of his letters to Rhine (dated March 21, 1949), at the time serving as the director of the Duke University Parapsychology Laboratory, Schulze reports having asked the family for permission to have the adolescent stay with him at his premises, to directly witness the strange phenomena that were surrounding the adolescent, as reported by the family.

There was an important case in 1949. Do you remember this case? Can you tell me a little more about it? What happened?

Schulze: There is no more to say. [Although he had previously told me that he was going to talk about the case, suddenly he surprised me with his initial response, getting back on topic in the questions that followed.]

Oh, I see. So, do you know what happened to the family?

S: I think the mother is dead, the boy says he doesn't remember anything about this.

Oh, he doesn't remember anything. Is he still alive?

S: I do not know.

And what exactly did you see on that night?

S: We had twin beds and his bed began to shake. [In the letter to Rhine, Schulze reported that the bed shook whenever he was on it. There was, however, no apparent motion of his body.] Next, I asked him to get out of the bed and lie on the floor, and he got on the floor on the rug, then the boy and the rug moved. [In the letter he writes: "I made a bed on the floor for him and this glided over the floor."] I asked Ronald, "Are you doing this?" And he responded, "I am not doing this thing." Also, he sat in the chair, a very heavy chair and the chair turned over.

Really. Wow. So, were you able to stop the chair from moving?

S: I did not try. So, let's see what else…. I think he laid down on the floor and he went to sleep. I wanted to put him in the hands of a doctor who would be sympathetic to the case and his parents wouldn't let me do it.

But do you think there was something happening, like some sort of spirit activity that made these things happen?

S: Something very serious was happening, the family doctor not getting the parent's consent to put him in the hospital. I forget the city they were from in the west. [In the letter, Schulze wrote that, although they did not allow the doctor to hospitalize the boy, Schulze convinced them to place the adolescent in the hands of Dr. Mabel Rose, a physician from the University of Maryland. She and her staff interviewed the boy twice. He was supposed to have gone for a third appointment.]

Okay, according to this report, they were from some city in Missouri—St. Louis, Missouri.

S: Yes.

Was the name of the family, the Hunkeler family?

S: Yes.

And how old was the adolescent when the events happened?
    S: About 14 years old.

Where is he from?
    S: American.

How did he look physically?
    S: [no response]

Accordingly, there were some marks that appeared on his body, some that the doctors inspected [caused supposedly by the possessing entity]. What kind of marks were they?
    S: Let's see. I didn't see any marks like the ones the family reported, but apparently from what the family said, there was a red mark that was upside down on his body. I thought that he did this to himself. [Some marks appeared on the body of the adolescent, spontaneously, and yet when Schulze and his personal doctor examined them, he wrote to Rhine that they looked more like psychosomatic rashes brought on by nerves. Schulze wrote, "Words also appeared on the boy's body, according to family and friends. My physician and I saw no marks, but we did see nerve reactions, which had the appearance of scratches." These marks on the adolescent's body supposedly indicated to the family that they should take the boy to St. Louis. From a dermatological and scientific standpoint, it is interesting to note that Schulze does not take what the family informed him for granted. He even separated what he believed from what was said to him, using the phrase "the family tells me." Also, he declared that he believed the boy did these marks to himself. The family claimed the marks constituted a complicated phase in the form of letters. Schulze did not see clear letters but marks that resembled nerve rashes.]
    [Note: In reports on the case, such as in Thomas Allen's book *Possessed*, the marks are repeatedly taken for granted as if they were real, as the most salient feature of the phenomena experienced by the possessed adolescent in this account of the case. In these descriptions of the Jesuit Report and the book *Possessed*, clear marks or letters appeared. However, none of the witnesses during the exorcism closely examined the marks; not even a medical doctor was called in to examine their nature. On the contrary, Schulze as firsthand witness clearly dismisses the appearance of the marks as not being clearly defined letters, but only scratches on the body of the adolescent. According to the definition of the word "scratch" in dictionaries, to scratch is "to break" or mark the surface by rubbing, scraping, or tearing with something sharp. In other words, Schulze described skin lesions that very likely imply a mechanical nature, such as the nails of the adolescent or an external device that may have caused them, thus dismissing the supernatural nature of these lesions or marks as legible and intelligible letters or words. Moreover,

it is important to note that stress causes a chemical response in the body, making the skin more sensitive and reactive. It can also make it harder for skin problems to heal. In some types of atypical dermatosis, marks in the form of lines can appear as one rubs the affected skin. The adolescent may have been undergoing deep stress, and under stress the skin becomes very sensitive.]

So, did you pray for him? Did you do something for him?

S: I had prayers for him and a circle of prayers was organized by some of the members of the church to help him out.... However, I don't remember all the details, after all this time, on exactly what happened.

But, returning to the matter of the moving furniture—you saw the chair moving?

S: Yes.

How big was the chair?

S: About the size of that one, where you are sitting.

Was it very heavy?

S: It was quite heavy.

How did it move? Backwards or how?

S: It moved against the wall as far as it would go and then took the edge and then turned around—with the kid sitting on the chair.

And where was it located? Was it in the middle of the room?

S: No, it was very close to the wall.

Also, did you say he was sleeping on the rug on the floor? You made him sleep on the floor because the bed was shaking?

S: Yes.

Did you sit on the chair yourself to see if it would move and if you could stop it?

S: No.

Well, then you saw the bed shaking, right? Did you take him out of the bed and make a bed for him on the floor?

S: I think so, then for the rest of the night he slept on the floor.

In one of the reports you mentioned that the rug started to move with the boy on it. And, so, what happened? What did you see there?

S: I saw the boy lying on the rug and the rug moving.

Where was the rug moving? Towards the wall? Was it going under the bed? Did you ask him, "Are you doing this?"

S: I don't remember after all this time all the facts.

And what happened afterwards? Did you take him to see some of your colleagues?

S: It was in 1949 and it happened to him during Lent. I called another pastor and told him about it. He said he couldn't come right then, so some time passed, and one of the other men did not respond in a timely way.

After what you witnessed at your premises, what happened to the adolescent?

S: Suddenly, the whole thing sort of disappeared. I lost track of it. There was a Roman Catholic priest who, as I understood it, served what they called a "black fast," where the priest doesn't eat anything during a period. He followed the order for an exorcism, the whole thing being sort of hushed up.

So, he had an exorcism? Did you participate?

S: No.

So, you brought over someone else to do it?

S: Yes, the Roman Catholic Church has denied that there was ever such an event, but they have a record of what happened. I don't know what they have done with it.

But did you talk to your superiors about the case?

S: I asked the Lutheran Church at that time and kept them informed, although I had no superior. The whole thing just disappeared. I heard on the report [Jesuit reports that Schulze had sent to Rhine] that he was taken to St. Louis and that some Jesuit priest performed the exorcism.

How long did it take place? Also, when he returned, was he free of the entity?

S: Yes.

Do you think he was really possessed by an evil spirit?

S: I don't know. It's hard to say. Sometime after that, the Roman Catholic Church denied that such a thing happened.

Did the family live in Prince George's County, Maryland? You also mentioned that the boy was put in the hands of the county mental health clinic, under Dr. Mabel Rose.

S: He's dead now.

And do you think that what happened that night was genuine?

S: Yes.

Do you think he was faking it or trying to do something?

S: The boy was not faking it.

Did you sense presence or some kind of strange feeling that night?

S: No, except that I wondered if I was going screwy.

I see, and what did you tell the family the next morning?

S: I told the family what I saw and I don't recall them doing anything about it. The boy had a favorite aunt in St. Louis and I thought that he wanted to go to live with this aunt, and he was doing this to live with that aunt. [Note: it seems that the family was initially convinced that Ronald was faking the phenomena to go to live to St. Louis.]

Was that what the family believed about the case?

S: Yes, the family claimed that the aunt of the boy—I don't recall exactly since it was so long ago—had some secret psychic ability or power that she could use to reach porcelain saints on a shelf. They were up too high for her and she had some way of getting these things down off a high shelf.

So, the family claimed that the boy's aunt had power and she was trying to make the boy go with her.

S: I think so.

Oh, I see. Do you believe that she was really doing something?

S: I don't think so.

Did you can talk to her?

S: I never met her.

But did the family believe that what was happening was real?

S: Yes, but there was also some type of deception and trickery occurring.

[Note: At this point in the interview, Schulze's wife Ruth entered the room and interrupted, explaining that Rhine and his wife Louisa had visited them and discovered on their own what Schulze had explained to them back in 1949.]

Ruth: Well, we had a unique experience with all that. The only thing that I remember is when Louisa came to our room and we had the sewing machine open, and she happened to hit a spool and a bobbin with thread on and this thing scooted out. I thought surely something was spooky about that! You know, the movie *The Exorcist* was based on an experience my husband had in our home, in a case that happened in 1949.

Do you remember the Exorcist movie? The movie was based on a case that he witnessed?

S: Now, stop it!

Whoa! [Laughter]

R: It is interesting that we meet you now.

Yes, I am very glad to meet you, you are very wonderful people. I am really enjoying talking to you. I am organizing all the documents that Rhine received on the case and we found this. I am planning to write an article on the Mount Rainier case.

R: Well, he just this day dodged interviews and questions about the whole thing, wanting to forget it—and I can understand why. Because we had these entire going-ons in our home, you know.

Did you witness any of these things happening?

R: Well, I was in the room next to these things occurring and I heard the racket and I knew the boy. I didn't see these things happen—right, honey?

S: Right.

Oh, I see. So, what was your impression of all these people approaching him and asking him these questions?

R: Well, all I know is he dodged it until this day, when people call up and want to have things explained and want to use his name. He doesn't want his name used.

No, I wouldn't do that. I am just organizing these materials for the Rhine Institute and to be used for my paper.

R: Is Mrs. Rhine still living? She has been there since the 1960s, right?

No, she died in 1982 and he preceded her, dying in 1980. Now the Foundation is under the direction of Dr. Ramakrishna Rao from India.

R: Oh, I see.

Can you tell me more about your impression of all these people approaching him and asking him these questions?

R: That was some experience I'll tell you. He never told me that before, he didn't want to talk about it and he wouldn't talk except for circumstances such as this one. In the case, we had the doctor in on it, and the family would never have the boy go to the doctor or the hospital, and even our doctor who wanted to be involved in it. They wanted the doctor to have no part of it. It was weird, I'll tell you.

What was the doctor's opinion on the case?

R: Well, I don't think Dr. Gray could decide on it, could he? He just refused to let him take part and have the boy go to the hospital, right, honey?

S: Right.

Did you meet this person named Richard Darnell? He was the president of the Parapsychology Society in Washington. [Darnell was familiar with the case and tried to convince Schulze to present the case before the society.]

R: We only knew Rhine through this experience, we had him in our home and, like I said, Mrs. Rhine came to our home one time. I had met the boy, but I didn't experience or see the reported events happening, all of this that was going on in our home. I could hear the racket; I was in the guest room while the boy was in the bedroom with my husband.

Was Ronald afraid of what was happening to him?
    R: Apparently not.

What else did they see? What was happening around this boy that you heard?
    R: We had prayers for this family—from the beginning of these happenings—and people who are living today experienced part of this. But when I want to say to people that *The Exorcist* was based on this experience, well, he gets mad at me.

Yes, it seems that, at that time, Blatty was going to Georgetown University and he heard the story from the news and then recreated the history and made changes and exaggerated the events. Did you watch the movie? Did you see the movie?
    S: I would not go to see that because I had firsthand experiences which I would rather forget.

Well, this is fascinating. Can you explain what happened, all the things that you heard about that were happening to the boy?
    R: I was in the next room and the racket was going on, he was on the rug on the floor, the furniture was tilted and all these rackets that I heard but I did not see it. He saw it.

What did the Rhines do when they visited you to investigate the case?
    R: Well, the only thing I can tell you is about that crazy thing that occurred when she came to see us: the sewing machine was open and she hooked into one of the bobbins and the bobbin and the thread went off. I thought, what is happening now? Just very weird.

What was Rhine's explanation about what was happening?
    R: You will have to ask the man, I didn't talk with Dr. Rhine at all. I met Mrs. Rhine when she came into our home and, you know, we have all the history written up in our synod office. He gave all that information to Dr. Orso. Right?
    S: Orso wasn't the Bishop at that time.

Darnell was president of the Parapsychology Society about 1949 or 1950. Did you give him a copy of the report?
    R: I don't think he gave anybody information except to the synod office, because pastors were inquisitive and called him about the details. So, he felt that this was part of the things that happened to a pastor.

I also heard, and according to the records we had about the case, that he [Ronald] was taken to St. Louis and they performed the exorcism there.

R: The whole family's name was wiped out from registry from this area because they didn't want it published as history. They didn't want any part of it as recorded experiences so we don't know what happened to the boy.

Are they still alive, do you know?

R: No, and I don't think anybody from that church would know either.

Also, I heard that there was a press release.

R: They had it in the paper but they had all the facts mixed up, right, honey?

Who gave the press release? Did you give it?

R: They tried to get it from my husband but they didn't get any information. They picked up parts of information, although not from him, because he wanted no part of it. After they moved, the case was closed as far as we were concerned.

You must have had a lot of pressure from the press at that time.

R: It was terrible. It was awful. They really plagued him with telephone calls and all of that kind of stuff and he wanted out of this, we had had it. Is this part of the university's information?

Yes, I am organizing the archives on the case at the Foundation for Research on the Nature of Man and I am interested in all of the reports and documentation on the Hunkelers' case.

R: Well the synod office would have that, right?

S: I don't know.

R: Well, you gave it to the synod president, right?

S: OK, the Maryland synod, and I also sent a copy to Rhine.

R: And that is on North Road in Baltimore, right? [This synod is an organization of pastors and churches. The address is 7411 Yogurt Road, Baltimore.]

So how could I ask for the report? Is there any way you could ask and get a copy of the report for our archives?

S: Well, I think that what you would have to do is talk to the present synod president. However, that is access and information they are surely not going to hand out easily. It is history as far as they are concerned and they are not going to relinquish that information easily.

Nurse [just coming in]**:** My God, that is interesting and they never even told us! I'm not coming into your room at night any more. I'm not even coming down that end of the hall anymore. It is amazing how such memories come back!

S: I couldn't forget that, believe me, the first persons we told this to was a preacher we had lunch with and he couldn't believe it.

Where is the church located now? I couldn't find it.
　　S: St. Stephen's is on Redwood Road, off Rhode Island Avenue 18th, there is a church there, an African American church now. It is very inconspicuous—they tried to hide it from the public. It is on a hill but you can't hide anything on a hill.

Is that the downtown area?
　　R: Yes, in this area, northeast.

So the church is still there? I asked the operator and she said that she did not have it listed.
　　R: Why don't we send him down to Ida Mae, she'd really be able to talk to him, wouldn't she? Her name is Ida Mae Donley, she works here on Thursdays and she is down in the sewing room. She may be down in the sewing room this afternoon since this is Thursday. The sewing room is down in the basement all the way down past the cafeteria. She was part of the prayer experience and we had prayers over all this.

Did she witness something? I heard that Denis Brian interviewed Rhine several years ago and specifically ten years ago, about the case. He wrote a book about Rhine—a biography, The Enchanted Voyager.
　　R: He didn't give interviews to anyone about this, if he could help it.

Oh, really? So who was the last person he talked to about it, do you remember?
　　R: Someone by the name of Pfeifer in the Washington, D.C., area.

Was Pfeifer one of the pastors?
　　R: He died, and the man who was pastor at St. Paul's here, what was his name? He married Betty's sister, Linsky. He was as involved in this as you [Schulze] were, right? Not Linsky, but another preacher that wanted you to give him information.

What did Donley witness?
　　R: I don't think she witnessed anything that we experienced, as she was part of the prayer group. You see, all of this happened in our bedroom and our guest room.

Back to the question: Did you experience something strange in the house?
　　R: All that I knew then was that I heard this racket, and I was aware of what happened and what my husband was going through.

So did you talk to somebody else about this?

R: No, as I said, he never wanted to talk about it to anybody, let alone the press, because they could get things all screwed up and he had to protect the family and what they were going through. You see, this boy was an only child.

You haven't heard anything about him anymore?

R: Oh no, I think they moved out of this area and I don't think anybody knows where they are. The Catholic Church picked this up. The Catholic Church picked this devil thing up and worked with him over the years and they have taken credit for having eliminated this thing—whatever it was.

S: True.

Can you please clarify?

S: They claim that this priest did a black fast and that the priest lost so much weight during the fast that they put a statue of St. Michael in the room of the boy. This is all hearsay and after it all happened. This is what transpired as far as the Catholic Church is concerned. I wouldn't be a bit surprised if a Catholic publication had all this history, right?

Could be, so what did you decide to do? Did you try to get him linked to a doctor?

S: You see, our family physician wanted the family to put this boy in the hospital and they would not consent to that because of what happened here. I recall the family called in a woman, who did some kind of spirit anointing. I remember now, this woman folded a piece of paper and it opened up, some kind of ruse. She took a piece of paper and folded it tightly and it would open up. I did the same thing with a piece of paper and it would open up, too. So she was trying to prove that she had powers. She saw the boy and was in the home at the same time I was there. I said, look, I can do the same thing with the paper, and so I think she thought I stole some of her thunder.

So, actually, you did the same thing she did? She was trying to prove that she had powers by trying to tie the paper and you could do the same thing. So how would you do it with a piece of paper?

S: Just roll a piece of paper tight and it opened up.

And so she said she had powers because she was able to do that and you replicated it? And what did she say afterwards?

S: I said, "Look, I can do the same thing." And she thought I had taken away some momentum.

But how did she feel about it? Did she like it?

S: She didn't like it.

R: There are so many details that you forget over the years.

So she went to see the boy and what else did she do for him?
R: I don't know anything about that, it is so long ago and I don't know the details.

And how did they do with the prayers?
R: We had the prayers, because we thought we needed God to guide the family since they wanted no part of the hospital or doctors. Let me find out if Ida Mae is downstairs.

This is very interesting, I'm glad you still remember most of the details of what happened.
R: It is amazing because he wants to forget the whole thing.

When Rhine visited you, what did he do in the room?
R: Mrs. Rhine was there but I never met him. Would you please ask Rodell if Ida Mae is here today?

What did she do in the room?
R: I don't remember, except for that crazy thing with the bobbin that shot thread all over the place. I was sure that was part of the spooky thing that was happening.

Then what did Mrs. Rhine say about it?
R: I don't remember.

When was the last time that you talked about the case?
R: I am going to let you go down to the sewing room. I have a hair appointment now. You [Schulze] have a foot appointment too; he has to go somewhere too.

Well, I really appreciate all the information that you have given me.
R: You haven't got much from me.

What is your husband's reaction after all these years?
R: He just took it in stride; he is a very stable yet unemotional person. It is just part of the happenings when you are in the ministry, but it doesn't happen very often.

But do you think that he really believed that something of a spiritual nature was happening?
R: I have often asked him how he can explain the occurrence and he can't, it is one of those mysteries.

That's part of the report in 1949. You see, Rhine was in parapsychology at Duke University and that was the man that was contacted by your husband.
R: I still don't know who did.

So what happened with the press? Did they give you a hard time?

R: Well, they just bugged him every chance they got and they got the facts all mixed up. He wouldn't give them the name of the patient because he wanted to forget it.

Has he had someone visiting him recently about this?

R: No, look at the fact that the nurses didn't even know about this.

How old is he now?

R: The 30th of this month he will be 85.

How long have you been married?

R: Almost a century, we have been married since 1932 or 58 years.

Did William Blatty interview or talk to him?

R: No, this is the only time we have stated that there exists any relationship between what happened and the film, *The Exorcist.* We knew from what we had heard about the movie that it was based on this story. I also understand there was a girl portraying Ronald in the movie.

So did you hear anything else about the Jesuit priest who performed the exorcism?

R: As far as we were concerned, this was something that was just unpublished. I don't even know how we got the word that it was terminated, but I do know that the family moved out of this area.

Did you watch the movie?

R: Oh no.

So who told you about the relationship between the case and the movie?

R: We just put it together, because it was so closely aligned with what really happened.

Of course, I am sure that a lot of the facts in the movie were manufactured by Hollywood writers. I was really surprised when I watched the movie many years ago. As I watched the movie for the first time, I noticed that it was presented in such a way so that people would believe it was being depicted accurately and on a real case. However, I thought that they had exaggerated. I didn't find out about the actual facts until I came to work at the institute and found the actual story. I thought that it would be a very good idea to have all of the completed reports on the case.

R: You are very lucky that he would give you the information that he gave you. Yes, he has been reluctant to give out the information, but he knows that it is history.

So who would be the best person to talk to about this case besides you?
R: Ida first, and then try to get the report from the synod [Lutheran Church].

What happened to the physician, your personal physician?
R: He died.

And what did he think about all this stuff?
R: He was a very private and reserved person and I don't think, if you would have talked with him, that he would have made a commitment any more than my husband would, in explaining what happened.

Did he witness something?
R: You see, he was the one who tried to get them to consent to take the boy to the hospital for study or for information, but the family would never consent to anything like that. For example, there was no plausible explanation for the way that things which were hanging or shelved on the wall would fall down unexplained.

That is very interesting.
R: So, he actually told me about what happened; that the boy was sleeping on the bed and that the bed was shaking, the chair turning over and in every position that they were in, it was changing and banging and I heard it loudly from next door.

So where was your house located, in Washington?
R: We lived at that time on Barnum Place in the Northeast.

And that is where all that happened at that house?
R: Yes.

Is the house still there? How does it look now?
R: We rode by it years ago and it looks about the same. They are grouped homes and we were in one of the houses on the end. They were new during the war and a lot of army people lived there. He [Schulze] was a chaplain during World War II.

Is it like a complex of apartments?
R: No, they were group houses.

Let me see if I have anything else to ask you about this. So, who was Mr. Edwin Hunkeler? Was he a pilot?
R: Yes, that was the family name.

Do you remember Mr. Edwin Hunkeler? The father?
R: We knew the whole family; they were members of our church.

How did he react to this?
R: [No response]

You say you don't remember Dick Darnell, right? How many members of the family used to go to the church?
R: It was just that little family, he was an only child; there was the father, mother, and the child, Ronald.

So how did the family approach your husband?
R: He was always a very good pastor and, of course, when they had this problem they called on him and this is how we got involved, through the pastoral relationship to the family.

And then did he visit them? Did he go to their house?
R: I have no idea. I guess that he called on the first person that he thought could help—and that was our doctor.

What did Ronald look like?
R: A normal teenager, clean-cut kid. They were a nice family.

Do you know if he was afraid of what was happening? How about the father?
R: No, I don't really know what his reaction was.

So was the house in Cottage City, Northeast Washington?
R: Yes, we were near the church that we served—on 18th and Barlow Ave.

So, where you lived, was it close to the church?
R: About a mile and a half from the church.

And how about the family's house?
R: I didn't know anything about their home or its location.

Is Cottage City a town?
R: I couldn't find it on the map. I would say that it is a town in Maryland but am not sure. The church was close to Rhode Island and 18th and we were on South Dakota Avenue. It is very well-known, not hard to find. We will go now and I will try to find Ida Mae, the person that I told you about. She knew the family from church, a very nice woman.

May I take a picture with you and your husband?
R: What would you want that for? [She declined having her picture taken.]

For my own personal collection.
R: Ida Mae says that it was through her that the family first learned about the church. I got to know them through the Parent-Teacher Association

of the school (PTA). You see, I had children that attended the same school as the Hunkelers. The Hunkelers were active in our PTA. I had no contact at all with the boy when he was having problems. The parents had come and asked me for help because I was the closest one to them, in the church at that time. They asked me what they could do or where they could go. And having known that I was from Pennsylvania—and the Pennsylvania Dutch knew and believed in "pow-wowing." Are you familiar with the term?

No.

R: The person who did the pow-wowing was supposed to have power, asking for deliverance and healing in the name of the Holy Trinity. But they did it through prayer and that's how the pow-wow was done. More than that I don't know.

So what did they tell you the first time they asked you about it?
R: Well, they were having problems and they didn't know what to do. They had him see medical doctors and everything else. They were trying to get ahold of every resource that they could find in order to get some relief for the boy.

What did they tell you about what was happening?
R: Things were moving; things would fall off the wall or fall over when he was in the room. These same things were also happening in the boy's home. They took him to our home and the same things happened there, so they knew it was not something in the building itself and, instead, that it was coming from the child himself. In regard to the pow-wowing, I remember when I was a child that they would get information about some infection and these healers would go and pow-wow, laying their hands over the person and saying a few words. You never knew what they were saying, it was a silent prayer. I know they used the blessed name of the Holy Trinity.

So, they practiced some kind of ritual on the boy?
R: Yes.

By doing that ritual what happens? Does it visibly help the person?
R: Well, if the person has faith and the actions heal them, they might believe that is what did it. I am not sure if this is what actually happens.

You said that you did form a prayer group, at the church.
R: We all got together and prayed for Ronald, while this thing was happening. Mr. Hunkeler himself, he was a Catholic to begin with and had changed his faith to the Lutheran congregation. He left the Catholic Church and had become convinced that they were being punished, in some way, through the affliction of Ronald. Finally, the last thing they did was to contact a Catholic priest of some kind and this priest took the child and performed

the exorcism ritual. The Hunkelers, at that time, promised that if the boy would be cured that they would go back to the Catholic faith. And they did take the boy to a session in the Midwest somewhere, and they got their exorcism, whatever that consisted of. I never saw the movie based on this story. So, you are writing a paper on this?

Yes.

R: If you write a paper send us a copy.

I can send you the information in these papers.

R: They [members of the nurse staff] said that if you were going to write something we should get a copy.... Getting back to the story, after that, they say he was cured by the priests and the Hunkeler family rejoined the Catholic Church, after that losing track of the family. The father joined a Masonic Lodge later. The boy was cured and grew up and got married, that being the last I heard of him. The Lutheran Church building is still there, but it has been remodeled now.

Finally, after I completed the interview with the Schulzes, Ruth gave me the directions to the church (where Schulze was a pastor), indicating that the church had probably changed to a Baptist church. She sent me downstairs to the volunteers' section; there I was introduced by a nurse to Ida Mae, who was at the moment at the retirement home. Ruth had already phoned Ida downstairs, and had informed her about the reason for my visit to the retirement home.

As I greeted her, I saw a group of women, probably in their late 70s. Ida looked at me and said, "All these people were members of St. Stephen's where Reverend Schulze was a pastor. All of us have followed him here since he retired as pastor and continue to be loyal to him. Most of us were members of the circle of prayers that was conducted in aid to Ronald Hunkeler."

Next, we got into Ida's car and she took me to the places where the events had taken place. First, the Hunkelers' home, which was close to the school the boy attended as an adolescent. She also took me to the house of the Reverend Schulze, where the adolescent had spent the night at the premises. As she took me around the small town, she told me stories about her experiences as one of the best friends of the Hunkeler family. They were part of the same school organization, used to have lunch and breakfast together, and had introduced her to the Lutheran Church. Also, Mr. Hunkeler was really skilled in carpentry work and had made some nice wooden earrings for her. (She allowed me to take a picture of the nice earrings.)

Appendix C
Interview with Ida Mae,
the Leader of the Circle of Prayers

Once I completed my interview with the Schulzes near one of the nurses' stations, I thanked them and was then directed to one of the main sections of the retirement home, where the volunteers used to join and work most of the time. As I walked downstairs, I saw a group of women, most of them in their mid-seventies, talking about and planning the volunteer activities for the day. I was then introduced to Ida Mae, who had been the main organizer of the circle of prayers that were conducted at the Lutheran Church. Once we completed the tour of the places where the events had taken place in 1949, Ida invited me to have coffee and speak about the case, allowing for an interview for the first time in an informal manner.

The Circle of Prayers

In a very solemn manner, Ida handed me the phone stating, "Okay, you wish to talk to the real Ronald, the one on which the movie *The Exorcist* was based? I will put you on the phone with Ronald. His family and I have been very close friends since 1949, we belonged to the same church, since those years and maintain up to this time a close friendship." As far as Ida knew, he had never talked to anybody outside of those involved in the case, since it took place, such as the priest who conducted the exorcism and some of us who were part of this ordeal. After ringing him up, she briefly explained to Ronald the reason for my visit and the seriousness of the work I was conducting. Then she handed me the phone and said to me, "He will talk to you with the condition that you will keep his identity confidential." I was somehow nervous, introducing myself to him and revealing the importance and the seriousness of my research on the case for a book on the real story. Then, he replied, "I have never spoken to anyone about the case since it took place back in 1949, though I have received information about my story being the basis for a famous movie called *The Exorcist*. However, I never saw the movie and I would rather not talk to anyone about this issue, since I do not recall anything about what happened."

He continued, "My family and I have kept a low profile in this matter. Also, most of those involved in it promised not to reveal any information on the case. Even if I wanted to talk about it, I honestly do not recall anything about what happened. I am sorry that I can not be of much help to you. Please convey my greetings to our friend Ida. It has been nice talking to your, sir." Then Ronald hung up. Ida said, "I told you they prefer to keep this information secret. However, I appreciate your work and will provide you with some of the information that you need on the case and what I know about it."

Interview with Ida Mae Donley, 1993

Before conducting this second interview, I introduced Ida Mae to my findings on the Mount Rainier Exorcism case, my relationship with the Foundation for Research on the Nature of Man, and the initial details from my interview with Schulze and his wife. Ida Mae had been the organizer of the circle of prayers on behalf of the adolescent. I told her about my intentions to visit them again at the National Lutheran Home; however, she told me that the Schulzes were very sick now. She added, "I think he sleeps most of the time now and can hardly understand what is being said. Also, Ruth is in

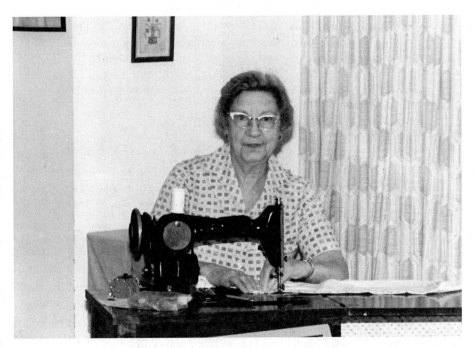

Ida Mae Donley, the organizer of the circle of prayers on behalf of Ronald (in 1993).

a wheelchair and fell on the floor and injured herself badly. I do not think is a good idea to visit them now. They are having too many health problems." Later in a letter, Ida Mae informed me that they both had died. However, now she offered to talk about the case for a taped interview. Ida was not only the organizer of the circle of prayers for Ronald; she was also a close friend of the Hunkelers, having met them through the school where her children and Ronald attended together in 1949. She had also been a personal assistant to Schulze when he was a pastor. It is important to note that this is a second, more formal interview and was a continuation of the informal interview that I conducted with her while she was driving her car to the places where most of the events took place regarding the Mount Rainier Exorcism. Back in 1990, shortly after I interviewed the Reverend Schulze, she took me on a ride in her old car from the National Lutheran Home to Mount Rainier.

It is important to note that the Hunkelers and Ida Mae were members of the PTA and met through this organization. She introduced them to the Lutheran Church and attended the services with them regularly. According to the recent obituary records that I obtained, she died at the National Lutheran Home at age 103, in 2009.

Well, I am interested in additional information on the case. Even though I got information from the Schulzes, I'd like to know more about it.
Ida Mae: As you know, this information is confidential like the doctor's information, they can't talk about it. For instance, if you go to a preacher you do not expect him to give you all the information you ask him.

Well, you know there is a book about the case from a writer, Thomas Allen. I brought a book for you to read; let me give it to you.
IM: Who is Allen?

He is a writer who wrote about the case, his book being more about the actual happenings and events that took place.
IM: Well, that is not your story, how about yours?

Mine is going to be more technical, about a scientific approach from a different perspective coming out of parapsychology and psychology. Did you know the boy?
IM: I knew the boy, he was younger. I showed you the school he attended.

Is the school still there?
IM: No, the school has been torn down, I showed you where the family lived and the school was right across the house. However, there is a community center where the school used to be.

How many brothers and sisters did he have?
  IM: None, he was an only child.

How did he look physically?
  IM: I think he was okay, as far as I knew he did not have any physical problems.

I mean, how was his physical appearance?
  IM: He had white skin.

How did you get to know about the case?
  IM: The family and I worked together in the PTA and joined our church. They came from the St. Louis area, putting their son in the same school as mine.

I learned that they were Catholic and then became members of the Lutheran Church.
  IM: Whether the boy was baptized Catholic, that I do not know; I know Mr. Hunkeler was baptized Catholic but I do not know about his wife. Her mother lived with her for a while. Mr. Hunkeler had given up the Catholicism and at the PTA they asked about a church and I told them about the Lutheran church in our town. Soon after, they began attending our church.

How was your relation with them?
  IM: We were very good friends and worked together, they were active in PTA projects at school. In our church, she joined the women's group and we used to have dinner together. They always participated and were big supporters of such activities.

How about their personalities?
  IM: Very social.

Were they very strongly attached to the church?
  IM: They were regular churchgoers, they participated in the activities. However, when they began to have the problems they came to me since I was from Pennsylvania and of course there are these people called the Powai. They were looking to every source for help. They wonder if I knew somebody who would do Powai. I knew somebody but I did not recommend them for that.

What is the Powai? Is it like a healing system?
  IM: You know there is a group of people that use the Christian Trinity—the Father, the Son, and the Holy Ghost and they do this kind of Powai healing. They were thinking that maybe this method could help them some way.

Were you the first one they approached about the case?
　　IM: That I do not know.

What was the first thing you heard about the case?
　　IM: He was having problems; they were having problems and funny things were happening.

Did you know if they were interested in strange things such as the Tarot or occult practices, etc.?
　　IM: That I do not know. Suddenly we kind of lost track of the family.

What else comes to your mind after all these years that you can recall?
　　IM: Well, Mr. Hunkeler rejoined the Catholic Church, St. James Catholic Church specifically. He thought that he was being punished with the problem because they had left the Catholic faith. Also, when they took the boy for an exorcism they promised God or the Saints that if the boy would be cured they would return to the Catholic faith.

And they actually returned to the Catholic Church.
　　IM: Yes, they did. They returned to St. James Church. Mr. Hunkeler was also a Freemason; he belonged to the Masonic Lodge over in Mt. Rainier. My husband and Mr. Hunkeler were members of the same Masonic Lodge.

What kind of organization is that? Is it like a religion or philosophy?
　　IM: Well, a lot of people have taken it as a religion; however, it is a secretive fraternity. Some people have joined that instead of practicing a formal religion.

I am a little tired; can I have a glass of water?
　　IM: Certainly, and let me show you something Mr. Hunkeler did for me for my birthday one year.

What is it?
　　IM: Look at these beautiful earrings made from wood. Mr. Hunkeler had made them for me. He was good with his hands, working with wood and with electrical work, etc. He refurbished some of the carved doors of our church.

They look very nice. So he used to do all kinds of work on wood?
　　IM: Certainly, he knew how to work on all sorts of wooden furniture. He was an able carpenter, used to also do plumbing work for the church and our house.

Appendix D

In the Grip of What?
Interviews with Experts
on Demonic Possession

This appendix includes the complete interviews with some of the experts on demonic possession who participated in a documentary about the Mount Rainier Exorcism, titled *In the Grip of Evil*, produced by Henninger Media Services, Inc., in 1996. This film constitutes the best scientific documentary ever produced on the Mount Rainier Exorcism, which reveals the most accurate and reliable information on the true story behind *The Exorcist*. I was invited to participate in this documentary along with other international experts in the areas of diabolical possession, religion, and science, and the director of the film *The Exorcist*. These interviews are included to provide the reader with some complementary information to better understand the phenomenology of demonic possession and exorcism in the context of the Mount Rainier case.

Also, I include these interviews to expand on what was already said by some of the participants in the documentary, as well as on some related complementary topics on demonic possession and exorcism. The interviews were provided to this author by one of the directors of the documentary as reciprocal support for the author's book, in return for the information provided by the author to produce the documentary. As they were provided by Henninger Media, they appear as they were sent to me unedited. I have included a title for each of the interviews based in the general or main topic addressed by the experts interviewed to facilitate the comprehension of the interviews. Finally, I include a brief biography of the participants at the beginning of each interview.

In the Grip of Evil is a sixty-minute documentary that explores the issues of exorcism and demonic possession and its meaning as of the late 20th century. Leading experts in the fields of psychology and theology face off in the classic battle royal of science versus religion and good versus evil.

Does the Devil Exist? Jeffrey Burton Russell, Ph.D.

Interview conducted on September 30, 1996.

Russell is a well-published American historian and religious studies scholar. He is currently Professor Emeritus of History at the University of California, Santa Barbara. He is most noted for his five-volume history of the concept of the Devil: *The Devil* (1977), *Satan* (1981), *Lucifer* (1984), *Mephistopheles* (1986) and *The Prince of Darkness* (1988).

Does the Devil exist?

Russell: Okay, okay, does the Devil exist? The Devil certainly exists historically. Yes, the Devil exists in the belief of many religious traditions, including the Jewish tradition, the Christian tradition and the Muslim tradition. Figures of evil abound in different other traditions such as Buddhism. But only in the three Western traditions, Judaism, Christianity and Islam, is the Devil seen as an immensely powerful force that is countervailing to God. I should add Zoroastrians; that is another religious tradition where he is important.

How was the devil perceived in the past?

R: Well, in the custom, in literature, the Devil was a vague kind of figure. He was known as Satan, which means the "obstructing spirit" or the "obstructer," the one who gets in the way. And various individuals are called Satan in the Old Testament. It doesn't necessarily refer to the prince of evil, but just to somebody or something who is obstructing the right way. Along about the first century B.C., in the period of what is called Jewish Apocalyptic Writing, there the Devil fully emerges as Satan, fully emerges as the prime enemy of God. This great spiritual figure, he was an enemy of God and an enemy of all that is good. And then Christianity, in the first century A.D., takes over from that first Jewish Apocalyptic tradition, and then the Muslims later draw from the Judeo-Christian tradition. And so, Satan or Iblise is a big factor for them as well.

What role does the Devil play in the Bible?

R: Well, the Devil plays a very important role in the New Testament, and Jesus—one of his prime functions is to do battle with the Devil, to drive him out of people's lives in one way or another by converting them by moral suasion and that sort of thing. Other times, of course, Jesus is sometimes faced with the Devil in a more direct fashion. When he goes out into the desert by himself and is tempted by the Devil for forty days and forty nights. Other times, of course, he encounters people who are possessed by the Devil and then he cures them by commanding the Devil to leave these possessed persons. What we would call exorcisms. I'd say that the role of the Devil in the first few centuries of Christianity was immense. It was a period that for three or four hundred years in which people keenly felt the presence of the Devil right near them, right at their side tempting them and invading their minds and so forth. And one of the great movements for early Christianity was the monastic movement. They moved out of the cities into the desert so the people could become hermits or monks. And one of the things they thought they were doing was going out to fight the Devil, to struggle with the Devil in the wilderness.

How about the Devil of the Middle Ages?

R: Well, we don't like to use the words "Dark Ages." It's an old-fashioned word [for] the Middle Ages because it wasn't a dark period in any significant sense. The Devil is still a fundamental point in Christian doctrine, although the Devil has never been defined as a dogma in the Catholic or the Orthodox Church, or as far as I know, any other major church. But, nonetheless, the belief in the Devil is theologically accepted or acceptable. It is clear in offhand remarks and offhand comments by bishops, popes, [and] councils, who assume that the Devil is existing. They don't make an absolute statement that he does, but the assumption is that he does. Now, he becomes gradually, after the first three or four centuries, less immediately present. People still believe in him but there is less of a sense that he is around everywhere or waiting to get at you at every moment.

Has the belief in the Devil disappeared in the 20th century?

R: Yes, that is an interesting question, because although the Devil fades for hundreds of years, I don't mean disappears but becomes less important. The Devil begins to be more important, again, in the fifteenth and sixteenth centuries and the Protestant reformation struggle between the Catholics and the Protestants in Europe in the sixteenth century, was a time when the belief in the Devil was revived and perhaps stronger than it's ever been since the first centuries of the Church. Martin Luther, for example, made an enormous point of the Devil; he said that he had seen it and that the Devil had attacked him on numerous occasions. He had all kinds of advice for what you do when the Devil is attacking you and so forth. It became very important.

Are there many references to the Devil during the Reformation?

R: Well, I would say that they were kind of caught up in the Reformation along with the Protestants in a heightened concern for the Devil, which declined gradually in the seventeenth century, and again it doesn't disappear. You see lots of references to the Devil in that period, but it is not as intense. And as you go to the eighteenth century, the age of Enlightenment, the age of philosophical logic and so forth and the beginning of what we call modern science and so forth, there is a tendency to back away on part of the Catholic Church, to back away from it, again not to say that he doesn't exist but just not to talk about it so much. Then, when you come down to the twentieth century, after the second Vatican Council, it's kind of passé now in most theological circles in Catholicism and Christianity and general people prefer not to talk much about the Devil.

How about the belief in the Devil in the Catholic vs. Protestant Church?

R: Well, there is a very little distinction in which the Protestants thought of the Devil and the Catholics thought of the Devil. If you do studies where people were accused of Satanism or witchcraft, of worshipping Satan, you know they appear just as much in Protestant areas as they do in Catholic areas. It's about 50–50. You can't say that Protestants did it more or the Catholics did it more; it depends on local geography. Some places were very intensely involved in terror of the Devil and the terror of witchcraft; in other places, it didn't seem to bother it at all.

How about possession and the Salem witchcraft trials?

R: Involving possession as such, well, of course you refer to the Salem witchcraft trials, which are probably the best known of all of them. Where these girls of the Salem trials, girls claimed to have been possessed by the Devil, which was called up by the servant or slave Tituba. And, as we know, they exhibited all kinds of symptoms of possession, for instance, frothing at the mouth and talking in incomprehensible ways. One of them throwing a Bible across the room and smashing it against the wall and so forth, acts like that. That's very famous, now, whether that is possession or not, of course, most modernists will give all kinds of sociological and psychological reasons for it instead.

How about the demons of the Devils of Loudon in a convent or monastery?

R: Yeah, that was definitely a Catholic phenomenon, the Devils of Loudon, where apparently, an entire nunnery, convent, monastery, whatever you want to call it, where most of the nuns were convinced that the Devil was loose. Some of them believed that they had sexual intercourse with the Devil. They were shouting obscenities and were completely out of control, I think. We might say, again, how do you look at something like that? Again, from a scientific, historical, scientific point of view, you say that there was a priest who was accused of fulminating this, and actually acting as the Devil's servant and corrupting the nuns and so forth and he was executed. That's right.

Is there a consensus regarding the existence of demonic possession in the Catholic Church?

R: Well, I don't think that you probably can come together to a consensus; I think there's an effort on the part of theologians to move closer to a scientific point of view in this sense, that they are more and more concerned about the documentation of things like possession. And the general rule of thumb is that if you have an alleged case of possession, you look at it very carefully, and the first thing you look for is fraud. You know, is this person pretending to be possessed to get on television? Or is it fraud by somebody else? Is this person being manipulated by a wife, husband, mother, whatever, for that purpose? The first thing you look at is fraud, and if it doesn't appear to be fraud, then you look for a physical problem. Is this a strange disease, that physical disease that brings out these odd symptoms to the person? Well, if you've eliminated that, then you look for the psychological; is this person suffering from mental disturbance? And of course, it is at that level that you generally catch most cases of alleged possession. And then, there are some that aren't explained in that way. But I saw, I was at a conference at the Indiana Medical School where psychiatrists presented a videotape of a possession that was absolutely hair-rising. I mean, literally, I could feel my hair going up on the back of my scalp because it was a woman, a mother, a wife and mother, who would very occasionally start speaking in a male voice or at least a very deep guttural voice and cursing everybody in her family. I mean saying horrible things about everybody in her family. This was an evangelical family, so they called in a minister and the minister performed an exorcism or prayer service to expel the demon and she became temporarily better. But, a few days later, she became worse again, and the minister said, "Hey, look, I think maybe we'd better take her to a hospital and see what's going on." And so, the psychiatrist took over the case and with the family's permission, he filmed what was going on and it was absolutely terrifying. For instance, the woman would be sitting talking to the psychiatrist normally like this and suddenly she would arch over backwards in a way that you wouldn't think that a normal person could possibly arch backwards. Her head was just way in back and her mouth would open and these horrible guttural sounds would come out sometimes in Swedish.

Now, for a while, they were thinking, "What is going on here?" The psychiatrist finally determined, it's a long story, but he finally determined that she had had a grandmother, a Swedish grandmother, who had been herself suspected of witchcraft and apparently had done a lot of weird Swedish cursing around the family. And the woman had subconsciously remembered that, and at the point where she began feeling terribly guilty about something in her own life, all of this surfaced in her mind. There was a psychological base for that one, and if you had seen it, you would think, "Wow, this really is possession," but there was a psychological base.

Well, you see, the reason I said before that there is never going to be a complete consensus, is because we're dealing with two world views which are incompatible. From the scientific world view, you operate from the framework of the scientific world view; there cannot be any such thing as demonic possession. I don't care how many videos, how many things you can present, there cannot be any because such things cannot happen. Why don't they happen?

That's an interesting case of circular reasoning. Well, science can't deal with such matters and since science can't deal with such matters, they can't exist because the only things that science deals with can exist. It's very circular and it's very exclusive. So, science is never, no scientist, as a scientist is going to say, "Hmm, I guess you are right, this is a possession." They're always going to say that there is some act that you overlooked, some natural explanation you've overlooked.

On the other hand, the theologian is going to say—and it depends what kind of theologian, many liberal theologians would agree with the scientist. But more traditional theologians or evangelical theologians, and frankly from my point of view, more thoughtful theologians, will consider that this is a possibility. That there are reports in the Bible, that there are reports throughout the history of Christianity, some of them very well attested, and that these things may happen. So, you've got to be very careful in claiming one until you've done all the research to rule out everything else. But, when you've done all that ruling out, you've got something left, and then you're in a position to say, "Well you know, this could be, this really could be a demonic possession."

Well, I think the people who allow for demonic possession are right, that is a great problem and every society, even if society thinks that there is one truth that it lives by. If you were living in thirteenth-century France, you would be absolutely convinced that the entire Roman Catholic belief system was true. If you were living in twentieth-century Iran, you're going to be absolutely convinced that the entire Islamic world view is true, and so forth. We live in a society in the United States, which, curiously, most people are believers, but in which the leaders of opinion, namely my kind of people, academics, and your kind of people, the media people, tend to be very skeptical and very set in the scientific world view. And for those people, there is only that one world. There is only that one world view, so, if it isn't scientific, it isn't true, which, to me is illogical.

The twentieth century is, really, of course, one of the most horrible centuries that we've ever had. And I think what's happened to evil, I doubt that the actual quantity of evil or the actual power of evil has increased in the twentieth century. But I think what's happened, is the technology at our disposal is so much greater than a hundred or a thousand years ago. That we are able to make our own evil affect to affect so many other people in so many horrible ways. Stalin put to death 40 or 50 million people, so did Hitler, he wouldn't have been able to accomplish that much a hundred years earlier no matter how evil he was.

Are humans responsible for the presence of evil in the world?
    R: Well, I think that that is the interesting question. I mean, certainly humans are responsible for this and we all have within us a tendency towards

evil. We've all felt it one time or another and denying it, we've all felt the impulse to cruelty to hurt other people and hopefully, we repress it most of the time. But we've all felt it, particularly when we're driving on the freeways in Southern California. So, there is that destructive impulse within each of us, but what strikes me about the magnitude of evil, the evil of Hitler, or Stalin, or Pol Pot in Cambodia or these massive evils is that they seem to go beyond the evil impulses in each one of us. That is, if you took each one of us in this room together and added up all of our evil impulses, I don't think that we get anywhere near the kind of evil that we see. We wouldn't get anywhere near that proportion of evil, so it seems to me that evil is partly the responsibility of each of us as human beings. There also seems to be a transpersonal evil, again going back to the classic case of Nazi Germany, yeah, Hitler, you know, was an evil person, yes, but what about the millions of people who followed him? It went beyond the personal evils of these guys to massive evil. And it's, I've never seen a fully rational explanation for that, I mean you talk about mass psychology and mass psychosis.

Where does this evil come from?
    R: Well, okay, the next step on this argument is there a source of evil beyond humanity and we've talked about individual evil and collective evil, and then we're going to talk about something that goes beyond humanity. Is there anything in the cosmos that goes beyond humanity that is evil? Let's posit two things, let's posit first what we're used to doing in the twentieth century, extra-terrestrials; beings on other planets. Supposing these beings are hypothetical beings, have intelligence, we are also going to assume that those hypothetical beings have a choice between good and evil and will choose evil, so the evil is not just limited to the human race. In medieval terms, moreover, instead of positing extraterrestrials, the tendency was to posit angels, and there the theology was very clear that many of the angels chose evil and others chose good. So it's a phenomenon that goes beyond simply the human race into the other sentient beings in the cosmos as a whole.

Is demonic possession a superstition?
    R: To really believe in possession, without it being a superstition, that is, some people believe in possession without having anything to hang it onto. In order to have a coherent world view that includes possession, you've got to believe in the Devil or demons. And to believe in the Devil or the demons, you're going to have to believe in the wider picture that includes God and the creation of the world as something good.

What is demonic possession technically?
    R: Well, technically, demonic possession means that an evil spirit has entered a person's body and taken and pushed aside their will and their mind.

And so, it's now the demon operating inside that person rather than that person's own will and mind. Of course, there are some people who are very mentally disturbed and believe that they are possessed and believing that they can do horrible things to other people. "The Devil made me do it," except putting it in a real sense is frightening. You know, "the Devil told me to push my child out the window," or something like that. Well, a lot of harm is done in that way too. Of course if you tell, predictably, a child that they are possessed by the Devil, the child is going to act in ways that are very peculiar. I do not understand your questions on recent cases of reported possession. No, not really. I don't know. I don't think that anybody is calling everything in the world demonic possession; I don't think that they are talking about possession. What conservative Christians are talking about, is the influence of the Devil in the world and that can be possession, but probably rarely. More likely, it's just a suggestion, the temptations that the Devil offers people on a daily basis.

Why have you been interested in the topic of demonic possession?
    R: Well, my primary reason for doing it was because I had been, for a long time, fascinated with the problem of evil specifically in the context of the Judeo-Christian tradition. And the problem of evil is specifically how is there, in a universe created by a good God and ruled by good God, how can there be? Why is there such a thing as evil? I've learned that I can't answer the question, it's far too complex. It's far too beyond my powers as a historian. When I began working on this, I thought, "Well, I will treat this subject historically and examine all the things people have said, theologians and poets and so forth over the centuries." We may be able to pin down something about this, it's too complex, and it's too powerful.

In your opinion, what is radical evil?
    R: Well, radical evil is a term that sometimes I like to use instead of the Devil. When you say the word "The Devil" to people, most people think of a guy in a red suit with horns and a tail. Of course, nobody believes in that, so immediately people laugh and say that there is no such thing as the Devil. You don't use the word, "The Devil," but you think of radical evil and that is a root tendency on the part of human beings and perhaps other sentient beings, if there are some, to do evil. That innate destructive power we have in us. That is why I call it radical evil.

Is the devil just a church symbol?
    R: It's certainly not merely symbolic. It exists, it's a force. Is it a spirit or not? Again, you get trapped in what world view you use. From a Christian world view or a Muslim world view or a Jewish world view, it's a spirit. You better remind me, as long as we keep him under our foot or something like that or under our control.

How about William James and the Devil?

R: No, William James was a very practical and logical philosopher who was very interested in religious phenomena. And I think what he meant was that we are faced with the world practically, in which evil occurs. And there's no point in denying that evil occurs. What he was talking against was a kind of super-rationalism that we still have today. Where there really isn't such a thing as evil, as people being led astray, making mistakes or so forth, and he went on saying that it was very important to recognize the reality of evil. And, also, then we need to take the measures that are necessary to keep it under control in this world.

Did Sigmund Freud believe in the Devil?

R: Let's take one thing at a time, okay? Freud, of course, great genius, anybody would accept that he tended to be somewhat reductionist. He did not believe in any spiritual reality. He believed that all of religious experiences emerged from the human conscious and was really basically neurotic in its origin. So, for Freud, there's no Devil for Freud, there's no radical evil for Freud. However, there are psychological problems, sometimes deep ones that people have, which can be taken care of by psychoanalysis. Carl Jung is, of course, much more open than Freud in a variety of world views. Even more brilliant than Freud in that respect. He could understand that there are more realities than one. Also, Carl Jung took the Devil quite seriously; he took radical evil seriously in ways that were different than Christian theology, but nonetheless very seriously.

Is the belief in the Devil socially destructive?

R: If the Devil doesn't exist, then belief in the Devil is socially destructive. On the contrary, if the Devil does exist, belief in the Devil is a validity and necessity in trying to understand the control of evil in the world. Well, yeah. If you don't believe in the Devil, then what you encounter are people who are saying one way or another that the Devil made me do it. I couldn't control myself, it was some external force causing me to do this awful thing and, therefore, I'm not responsible, and of course that does happen. It happens to people having psychological problems, it happens to people in law courts, that kind of defense is used. So, there is a definite problem with shifting responsibility away from ourselves onto some other entity.

Is there any value in believing in radical evil?

R: The value in believing in radical evil is that, in my view, it's true that it exists, and if we ignore it, we are going to be caught by it in ways that are unexpected to us. I mean, if we start in the beginning of the twentieth century, it was a time of enormous hope. We had progressed, scientific progress, it was going to be a wonderful century, everything was going to be great and better and better.

What is the current image that people have of the Devil?

R: The original image of the Devil is, of course, a great fallen angel. And then, in the early Christian centuries, you've got the influence of art of pagan images, such as the god Pan so, by the time you get to the fourth or fifth century, it becomes more and more common to see devils with horns and tails and that sort of thing. Although sometimes you get some interesting variations of the Devil; he appears as a beautiful young person. The Devil can appear as any kind of color, blue, red and so forth. Sometimes quite attractive, but that kind of iconography of the horns and tails comes primarily from the Greek god Pan. It affects people differently at different times, some people, it clearly frightened. But I think that stereotypical picture of the Devil with horns and tails had lost most of its power to frighten people at least by the 1700s; and from then on, it became more and more as a joke.

Did the movie The Exorcist *increase our belief in the Devil?*

R: *The Exorcist* certainly revived interest in the Devil and probably increased belief in exorcism. There is a very powerful opening sequence in the opening in the desert where the dogs are howling, terribly fighting deities facing each other, and you have howling wind and so forth. This made an enormous impression upon some people and, personally, I know one person who actually went to a mental hospital after seeing the film, he was so deeply upset by it.

Why are we so upset about the Devil, about images of the Devil?

R: It reflects something in us, whether that thing is also outside of us. Whether the Devil exists outside of us, whether he is only inside of us, it depends. When we see figures, compelling figures of evil as we saw in the beginning of *The Exorcist*, we feel a deep residence of something within us and it frightens us sometimes to death.

Is there anything that frightens you about the Devil?

R: What frightens me, personally, is the Devil's influence, that is, the Devil is always around urging me to do things that I ought not to be doing. Well, I think that good and evil has been an interesting topic for people since the beginning of time. Why is there more interest now than perhaps 50–100 years ago? It is because evil has been so dominant on the international level. On the national level, the racial hatreds, all of that, and of course, the striking images of brutal crimes that we've witnessed recently. The Richard Allen Davis case up north, the case of the child abducted from her own home. The rape and murder of this child, we look at Richard Allen Davis and we have to ask the question, "What's going on in this man that causes him to do that?"

What is the source of evil in our society?

R: The source of evil, of course, there are many sources of evil and human society is one of them. Again, returning to Nazi Germany, this is an evil society which has evil fruits. It's also individual, and I don't think—one of the old sayings about the Devil is, "The Devil can't make you do it." That you cannot be controlled by the Devil if you don't want to be, and none of us can be controlled by anything evil if we choose. There's a moral choice that each one of us has, in any given circumstance, we can choose to do the good or we can choose to do the evil. In that sense, it is always an individual responsibility. And we can't blame it on the Devil, we can't say that the Devil made me do it. We can't say that my genetic system made me do it, we can't say that my parents made me do it, we can't rely upon any of these social expectations which are so common nowadays. There's got to be an individual moral choice at fault.

What is demonic possession and exorcism?

R: Possession is interesting, possession is involuntary. Remember what happens in possession is the demon sets aside your own intellect and your own will and acts in your body. Therefore, your own intellect and your own will are not corrupted by the Devil. Whatever that possessed person is doing, it's not his own intellect and will that is doing it. Therefore, when the Devil or demon, or whatever it is, leaves, the person's will and intellect is untouched.

What is the Christian procedure for exorcism?

R: Well, in Christianity, the process of exorcism is casting out a demon in the name of Jesus Christ. The idea is that the Devil is a powerful figure, a powerful spirit but that God is always more powerful than the Devil. Christ is always more powerful than the Devil. And so, in any circumstance where you can order the demon out of the person in the name of Christ, that is the way you get rid of the Devil, it's not that the Exorcist, himself, has any particular spiritual talents, although he may or may not have. It's the power of Christ that drives the Devil out.

Is exorcism common in other religions besides Catholicism?

R: Well, exorcism is very seldom performed in Judaism, certainly in modern Judaism. I don't really know what exorcisms are performed in Islam, although I know they occur. In Christianity, exorcism has been associated with, historically, the Roman Catholic Church and with the Eastern Orthodox Church. But we're finding more and more in this century, exorcisms being performed by Evangelical Protestants, and even some mainline Protestants, for that matter.

Why did The Exorcist *movie frighten people?*

R: Well, I think partly, we like to be scared by riding on a roller coaster, there's something in that, too. But I don't think that's all there is to it. I think we get a different kind of scare from watching a film like *The Exorcist* from the scare we get from riding a roller coaster. It frightens us because it's speaking to something deep inside of us. We have a sense that there is an evil inside of us that is being represented and is being brought out in this film, or this book, or whatever it is.

In your opinion, does the Devil exist?

R: Science defines itself in such a way that it cannot treat the question of whether the Devil exists. History, being a form of science and academic endeavor, history defines itself in such a way that it cannot investigate the question of whether the Devil exists. The problem is, whether natural science or history says it can't investigate that question, therefore, it doesn't exist. What they should be saying is that we can investigate this question. We can't have a judgment one way or another about it and many historians will say that, but most historians will go further and say that because it doesn't fit the boundaries that we've drawn for our own possession, excuse me, for our own profession. That's a Freudian slip because it doesn't, historians will say that because it doesn't fit the boundaries that we set for our own profession, it doesn't exist.

Is evil within us, as humanity?

R: We can learn the depths of evil within us, none of us wants to admit that. Everybody likes to think of themselves as good people. We like to think we're good people, and we're not just good people, we're a mixture. There's good in us, there's also evil in us, and one of the important things that Carl Jung has taught us is that if we try to pretend that we're good people, we tend to increase the power of the evil by denying it.

What is the origin of sin as evil?

R: Let me give you an answer that a very brilliant fourth-century theologian gave. He was a very good psychologist and he said that the origin of a sin, you know, an evil deed, lies within us. We open our minds to this, we start to think, "Hmm, I'd like to steal that person's car," or whatever it may be. And then he said, "As soon as we open up a little hole in our mind for that sin," he said, "then the power of the Devil rushes into us and expands us and tries to flood us."

What do you think about playing with the Ouija board?

R: We should be afraid in this sense: we should not play around with a certain, how you say, Ouija boards and that sort of thing. That's very frightening; I've seen and heard of some very frightening things about that.

Can the Ouija get us in contact with spirits?

R: Yeah. The Ouija board can be simply a parlor game; people aren't taking it seriously and so forth. The trouble is, people kind of get sucked into it because it seems to spell out different words. And then the mind begins to open up to whatever is out there, whether it is your own subconscious or other. I don't know, but then it can come up with some terrible, terrible frightening things. I know a young woman who was playing with a Ouija board and it started as a parlor game. They started getting answers, "Help me, please help me, I'm in trouble," and finally, she asked, "How can I help you? Where are you?" And the response was, "In Hell." Now that was largely emotionally disturbing to that young woman. Now, whether that was her own subconscious or was some other spirit we don't know, but it is very dangerous to open your mind to that kind of playing around. Good idea.

Will belief on the Devil vanish in the 21st century?

R: As we go into the 21st century, things are going to be different in the next century. We can't be sure that the dominant world beliefs we hold in our society now are not going to be dominant a hundred years from now. I can tell you that as a historian, because every age is confident that its world view is the correct world view. A hundred years from now, we are going to have a different world view. What that will mean in terms of beliefs in the Devil and so forth, I wouldn't dare to predict. The most important thing I can think of that we can do, is to open our minds to all of the possibilities that exist. Not to limit ourselves and stick to strictly the scientific world view, or stick to strictly a Roman Catholic world view, or strictly Muslim world view. But to open ourselves to other various possibilities that exist and to realize that reality is more complex than we think it is, and to realize that there are a variety of answers to most problems, not just one.

Is demonizing people or groups a real problem in our society?

R: Demonization is a real problem, Christians have demonized Jews, Muslims have demonized Jews, Jews demonized Muslims, and people with secular beliefs, they seem to be no less prone to demonize their enemies as people with religious beliefs. Demonization is a real problem, and if we stick to the basic religious principles which prevail in most world religions "Love God and your neighbor," there is a test we can apply. If I say that, oops!

Is demonizing people a form of evil?

R: Well, demonizing people is of course a great evil, and when people do it in the name of God, that is even a greater evil because it is blasphemous. And so long as we remember the essential point of all religious teachings, that is, to love God and other people, and we keep that in mind, then we won't believe that God is telling us to hurt another person.

How can we defeat evil?

R: I think the first thing we need to use is our discernment, that is our ability to tell the difference between good and evil so that when a thought occurs to us, before we act upon it, we need to discern whether that is something good or something evil. When another person comes up to us and suggests, "Let's do x or let's do y," then we need to discern whether that person is operating, basically under the rule of love or under the rule of hatred.

Can we do something to make this world better?

R: Yeah, you see, that's interesting, it reminds me of how—I'm not comparing myself to Mother Teresa, but it reminds me of an interview with Mother Teresa when the interviewer kept saying, "What can we do politically that will make the world better?" And she just said, "Well, we go out and help people. That's all we do."

But do you use your political influence to help people in need?

R: Well, we just go out and help people. Essentially, I think that—I don't believe that governments, that political movements of any kind are really going to make the world better. I think that it's up to us as individuals to choose to do the right thing and to obey the spirit of light as much as we possibly can.

Can you talk about evil and the Devil now?

R: I can't think of anything. I think that's a serious problem and even publishing my books run into this problem. When you talk about a topic like that, some of the people who are going to interested in it are going to be mentally on the edge, unbalanced one way or another. And they are going to be very upset about it, and you can't avoid that. So, yes, people who watch the television show are going to be very upset about this and to them, I can say, "The Devil can't get you unless you ask him to get you."

How would you define evil now?

R: So, what is evil? Evil is essentially the choice to do harm, to hurt another sentient being, to hurt a person or to hurt an animal, to hurt anything that can feel pain, to make a choice to do that is the essence of evil. Yes, and that urge to do evil is something that we all feel within us as individuals; the question is, "Does it go beyond the feelings we have us as individuals?" And it seems to me that movements like Stalinism in Russia and Nazism in Germany, the Khmer Rouge in Cambodia, and so forth indicate that it's not limited to individual evil. That it can be a desire that spreads through a whole large group of a population, the desire to hurt, to kill, to make other people miserable. So, it seems to transcend from the individual. Some people call it the Devil, you could call it radical evil, you can call it what you like, but it does exist.

The Nature of Evil: Father Dan O'Connell

Interview conducted on August 31, 1996.

Father Dan is a priest of the Archdiocese of Boston. He is currently pastor of Corpus Christi–St. Bernard Parish in Newton, as well as associate director of the Office of Worship and Spiritual Life located in the Archdiocese's Pastoral Center.

Is the church interested in the supernatural?

O'Connell: Well, because we are supernatural, we're interested in the supernatural because there is a part of us that transcends the day-to-day physical environment that we live in, and that is the spirit, and that is of every human being in this world. So our interests are in ourselves, and as St. Augustine says, "You have made us for yourself and our hearts are restless till they rest in thee." There is the interest, that's it, we're interested in the supernatural, the spiritual because we are spiritual, we're made for God, we're not made for this trivial everyday stuff.

Does supernatural evil fit in this world in the 20th century?

O: Well, it doesn't *not* fit. That is precisely the nature of evil: evil doesn't belong. Evil is something that comes into the world unannounced, yes, not announced, but unwelcomed. It's something that shouldn't be. The Scholastics used to call it privacioboni, a privation, a big hole in the wall. Something that shouldn't be there at all, and that's evil. Now it's evil in a spiritual sense for us. Evil is not something like the Empire State Building burning down; that's a derived sense of physical evil. The real horrible evils are what we call viciousness, hate, selfishness—the denial of all that we were really made for. That's evil. We're made for good. Satan, in the history of the whole Judeo-Christian tradition, is pure spirit, an angelic spirit, created by God, who failed the test of goodness definitively, he chose definitively evil, instead of good.

Do you believe in Satan?

O: Yes. The scriptures tell not that there is a Satan, but that there are hordes of evil spirits who went with Lucifer, failed the test, and were condemned to eternal hell. So they are the bad angels, evil angels. That's a strange term, isn't it? "Evil angels," nevertheless that's exactly what they are. I haven't seen nary a trace [of them]; these are part of our faith. That is to say, the whole system of revealed religion has this as part of its content; and by the way, it isn't the most important content. And that's one of the dangers in talking about all of this, the more you talk about stuff, the more important you make it, and these things are not as important as so many other things in the religious life of the human family.

When did you become interested in demonic possession?

O: Demonic possession came to my attention, historically, in the 1949 case. I had known about it theoretically in the writings of the Church, about exorcists and all of that, in an abstract way. It came into my life personally when I was asked by a young woman at St. Louis University to see a friend of hers, who had been told by three important Church people—let's leave it at that for now—that she was possessed, that the friend was possessed, so her friend came to me and said, "Father, will you see her?" And I said, no, I will not. First I would like to talk to Father Bill Bowdern because this is a matter that's very delicate, should not be engaged privately, or on one's own, and could cause a lot of trouble. For me, her, and perhaps other people. So I said no. And then I went to Father Bill Bowdern, and we talked about it. And that's where [I got] my knowledge, such as it is, very limited, very circumscribed by the whole setting, from my conversations with Father Bill Bowdern. The first thing he did was to tell me that I had been prudent in coming to him.

Did you read the Diary regarding Mount Rainier case?

O: He gave me the transcript of the 1949 case to read, and then he said, "Come back and we'll talk about it." And when we talked about it, we talked about what I had, secondhand, and of course, he threw me thirdhand, about the young woman who was in trouble. And we talked about whether I should talk to her, whether it would be prudent to talk to her, and after we had talked about the case, he said, "Go ahead and talk to her, I think that would be appropriate." And so I did. And what I thought was very brave was that the friend of the girl who had contacted me in the first place agreed to bring the girl with her, and sit in with her on her conversation with me, for the first part of it at least, even though I had warned her that if she was indeed—if the girl was possessed, that it could be a very traumatic, embarrassing, unpredictable situation. So she did, and I believe she sat in with us for perhaps a quarter of an hour, and then I said, "Karen, I think it would be OK if you leave, and let the young woman speak with me alone," which we did.

Also, at the end of the conversation, I told the young woman, "I don't think you are possessed, you're probably suffering from an eating disorder...." I'm not a clinical psychologist, by the way, so I don't diagnose, and I don't do therapy, and I'm sorry, but I think that must be made clear in my case. I'm just a simple priest who happens to teach experimental psychology. But I told her I thought it was clear that she had some sort of eating disorder, was probably depressed, and that she was not possessed at all. I heard her confession and sent her away and the only [further] contact I had with that young woman was through her friend Karen. And the report was that the young woman was very grateful, felt much better, much reassured, she had been scared out of her mind by the three people who, I'm sorry to say this, but I think irresponsibly told her that she was possessed.

Were you sure that she was not really possessed by the Devil?

O: First of all, if I thought she had been possessed, I wouldn't have pursued it at all, I would have referred her to Father Bill Bowdern and I would have pursued it. The signs of possession, however, are not psychiatric, and not psychological, per se. That sounds strange, I know, because a lot of people would say just that—I'm sorry, but I have to enter a demur. The original 1949 case was a perfectly normal young man, and, in fact, the reason that he was referred to the exorcist was precisely that the psychiatrist couldn't deal with him. Because the problem wasn't psychiatric, at all, and it wasn't psychological, at all, it was a problem of Evil.

How was William Bowdern, who performed the exorcism in the Mount Rainier exorcism, as a person?

O: Oh, a marvelous man, an old shoe, Irishman, and a storyteller. He was a pastor at the college church, St. Francis Xavier Church in St. Louis, for a number of years. And he was just a great guy, a quiet man, with a wonderful smile, and a very modest man. I had an eight-day retreat from him once as a scholastic, and he told—he didn't tell stories about the exorcism exactly, but he referred to it, adverted to it, and was very reserved about it. He did not talk about the exorcism freely or a great deal. I used to say that the one place in the country where the book and the movie were not discussed was the Jesuit recreation room at the St. Louis University, because Bill Bowdern wasn't keen on that, he didn't talk about it.

Was the case you read in the Jesuit's Diary a real case of demonic possession?

O: Yes, I'm quite sure of that from the transcript, which was of course his report to the Archdiocese of St. Louis. Well, I don't wish to claim that I remember all the details of that, but the gist of it was certainly that this was a genuine case of demonic possession, and that a genuine exorcism was needed, took place, and was successful. That was the gist of the entire thing, there's no doubt about it. On the other hand, and I think this is tremendously important, for the attitudes that have dominated this whole history in the interim, he told me this story. He said, "Dan, since that case, I have had over 200 referrals of people who were supposed to be possessed." In other words, he would, I'm sure, have gone along with what I'm about to say. That possession is not an everyday or even frequent occurrence, that it is extraordinarily rare, and that it is has nothing, per se, to do with psychological and psychiatric syndromes.

Was he an expert in demonic possession?

O: Well, the way he put it to me—again, he was an old shoe, he was not a theologian, and he didn't talk in theological terms. He said, "Dan, any seven-year-old could tell the difference between someone who is mentally ill, and someone who is possessed." Again, the point to be made, and it's not an easy point to make, that is to say it's not empirically easy to identify, although he did say "any seven-year-old." The difference between evil, viciousness, meanness imposed upon a human being, and mental aberration. They're two absolutely different things, they are not the same category at all. Now, obviously, when evil is impinging upon a human being from the outside, and that's the whole concept of possession, there is going to be some psychological effect. There's going to be some differentiation in the behavior of that person when under that influence, and their ordinary, normal, personal, responsible behavior. But that's another thing. The basic thing is to distinguish the two phenomena.

How is a demonic possession case diagnosed?

O: It's wonderful that the questions are posed in terms of sound and touch and smell and so on; those are relevant. They occur, obviously redeeming with someone who is embedded in the physical environment. Basic discernment of the exorcist is a spiritual one. It's discernment of good and evil, and it is the recognition of the presence of evil and more specifically of an Evil One, of a diabolical influence. There are details in the ritual of the Roman Catholic Church, but I would like to go back into the discernment of these, rather than the details. The basic point here is that there is something which is imposing upon a person from outside. That's why the unusual things are relevant, because these are the things that the individual, left to himself, doesn't do, cannot do, doesn't know about, and cannot produce. For example, the writing on the young man's back, this is.... I don't want to go into contortion. You can't do that sort of thing, it doesn't work. These are things that you're not capable of doing, the tremendous strength that he young man was capable of—a couple of the Jesuit scholastics did get injured in the process of holding him down during this process. All of that indicates something from the outside, not a condition of the young man himself.

Did the exorcists suffer any injuries during the exorcism?

O: No, the injuries that I hear about, and that were intrinsic to the transcript of the exorcism as it took place under Father Bowdern, were the injuries that the Jesuit scholastics experienced. And I, of course, knew those young men. Evil is, and there's a lovely German word for it, Erschreckent, ah, that's a great word. Evil is always terrifying, I mean real evil, viciousness. When we see someone being deliberately mean to someone who's vulnerable, we're all horrified, and in a sense terrified at the power that his evil has to destroy. We see it in a little child that's misused; we've had a lot of information about that. This week we've had the international conference on child abuse, the reason why we're so terrified by that, is because people are helpless, vulnerable, cannot be protected from this sort of meanness, viciousness, evil.

Did the exorcism performed by Father Bowdern affect his personal life?

O: Yes. Obviously, Father Bowdern survived and thrived for the rest of his life, he was not adversely affected in the long run at all. His faith was deepened, I know that, and he became, if anything, a more trusting man. Let me try to explain that, that's a paradox, I think, it sounds to me to be a paradox at the moment that I say it. One would expect that someone who is faced with the power of evil would be more frightened afterwards by the power of evil. That isn't the basic phenomenon. What Father Bowdern was confronted with was the power of God over evil. We do not live in a hobgoblin world, and that is the message that Father Bowdern radiated by his life. Not so much by individual words, he wasn't eloquent in any classical sense of the word, that old shoe concept comes back again. He was a happy, trusting, child-like man, and he was a very manly guy. So his experience, and the aftermath of his experience was a beautiful healthy increase, a child-like increase in his trust in God's power over evil. And the whole message of the exorcism, and indeed the reason why we can assume that God in his providence allowed it to happen, is very simple. In order to show the power of God, in his love all of us, over evil, evil doesn't win in the long run. And that is the message that this historic event was meant to communicate, and it was indeed a lived-happily-ever-after experience for the young man.

Did William Blatty ever interview Father Bowdern?

O: Absolutely not. The few mentions he made of this in his eight-day retreat that I made with a lot of other scholastics were typical. He was very reserved, very serious, and in no way melodramatic, simply by way of exemplifying a point for our retreat. He didn't talk about it a lot, he told me that when Blatty wrote to him, and this is certainly not verbatim, but the gist of what he wrote back to Blatty was, "No, I will not give you an interview, don't write the book, God bless you, period." Now, again, I don't have a copy of the letter. Bill Blatty can contradict that if he wishes, but in any event, that's what Bill Bowdern told me he said to Blatty, that he shouldn't write the book, that he wasn't going to get an interview with him, and that God bless you, I mean, "God bless you," was typical of Bill Bowdern.

Did Father Bowdern talk about the case with other members of the church?

O: Well, for example, I was at St. Louis through many of the years that Father Bill Bowdern was there, and to my knowledge he didn't give a lecture to the Jesuits on it, and so on. With hindsight you could say, maybe he should have. On the other hand, I think what he communicated was simply that this was a rare occurrence, that our attitudes toward it could be formed, if you will, from a distance, that we didn't need to engage it as a part of our everyday pastoral work. And, as he exemplified when I came to him, he was ready to help anybody that met such a case, but he didn't expect to meet cases, as he didn't expect to find cases in the over 200 that came to him. So he was not interested in some formal educational incorporation of this into the curriculum. [Interruption] Right, how to be an exorcist of the young seminarian. No way, and I think he was right, others would disagree with that, you have to arm people, as you say, you have to arm people to know what's going to come, um, hmm … no. there are other things infinitely more important that people don't learn anyway, so they should be learning these things.

Have we surrendered to evil in our society?

O: Always, to vindicate the power of God in producing well for that individual and for the world at large. We find that hard to understand, we find that hard to understand. Well, basically, we do not understand any physical evil that comes to the human family. The question is wonderful; we distinguish the horrible evil in people and the imposition of the evil from the outside by the criteria of what we are capable of. We are capable of a lot of evil, we don't need any help, now, we are warned by the scriptures that Satan does go about seeking whom he may devour, as a lion. That's the metaphor used, right? But from moment to moment, our inclination is to evil, and that's the doctrine of original sin, that our intellects are indeed darkened, that our wills are weakened, and that we have some inclinations that are really not healthy.

Do we have as humans an inclination to evil behaviors?

O: No, this … we can get some help from Satan in these domains, unfortunately, he can help in his usual "Screwtape Letter" manner. As C.S. Lewis pointed it out, "the devil is so smart," the best thing in the world for the devil is for all of us to deny his existence. Because then he can work as the prototypical espionage agent, who sabotages everything without becoming visible. OK, that's his ordinary procedure in the world. But most of the things that we do from day to day come from our own inclinations to evil; we're not entirely confirmed in goodness, to say the least. We're sinful folks, all of us are, we do mean things, we aren't very loving sometimes, and that's true of every single one of us, the Lord and his mother excluded.

Is the Devil in charge in this world?

O: I wish I knew. In principle, he could pick any one of us, but notice when we answer the question that way, we have to add immediately that he's not a free agent. He's not a free agent at all, his agency in this world; the limitations of his operation in this world are from God's own providence. It's God's world, we live in a redeemed world, not a hobgoblin world. And I have to keep coming back to that, the devil isn't in charge. "I'd like to choose Eleanor McGillicuty, all right, let's go." Ah, maybe, obviously very seldom, and under the providential super-ordinate control of a loving providential father. The father of this young man who was possessed is God, and he loved that young man more than his own parents loved him; that is what we have to keep in mind.

Does the providence protect us against the Devil?

O: I think the whole question of this—and I am delighted by Discovery's care to make this a serious, non-melodramatic and non-sentimental documentary. The whole point of contextualizing this properly is to contextualize it within the providential care of God. Our evil inclinations are countered by God's own grace and his influence in our lives, and we too are not, thank God, entirely free agents [interruption] we are protected. Our guardian angels protect us. God's providence protects us, and the intercession of the saints in Heaven protects us from ourselves, so that the psychotic who deliberately chooses, let's say, to seek, like a Faust, the cooperation of the devil, is not all that plausible. There's another agent involved.

Does God have a control over evil?

O: Let me put it as bluntly as possible. She's right, she's right, discussing these issues with mentally disturbed people can be extraordinarily dangerous. However, discussing almost anything with mentally disturbed people can be terrifyingly dangerous. Dr. Rappaport's problem is a very simple one empirically. We don't confront these cases, because they're so rare; of course she hasn't. Neither have I, and as an empirical scientist, as an experimental psychologist, my knowledge about this case and about exorcism in general is zero. As, and I would probably be saying the same thing as Dr. Rappaport, if I were wearing my empirical hat, I'm not, I'm not wearing my empirical hat right now, I'm speaking from my faith and the experience of my faith in a marvelous historical event. I say that deliberately, the winning out of God's providence and power over evil in this world, and that doesn't occur very often. God controls in it his wonderful providence that we don't understand either; and so, the psychiatrist who is working from empirical evidence, and has never met a case like this, is going to say exactly what Dr. Rappaport has said. Ask the psychiatrics that interviewed this young man. Ahh, there's another matter.

Do you think somebody can contact the Devil via the Ouija board?

O: Well, that's pretty standard. You know the Catholic Church has never been really enthusiastic about Ouija boards, for example, or any other games, séances, spiritualistic sessions that appeal to the spirits of the other worlds, as vaguely as they're usually presented in those contexts. So yes, that's something that one shouldn't play with. One shouldn't play with it, though even if there were no real danger of intervention, it's a silly thing to want out of, just out of pure curiosity to know than we mortals know. We're very curious creatures, we want to know everything, and that of course is one of our downfalls because we have to know everything and we insist on finding out. We don't like mystery, and mystery is so beautiful it should be retained, maintained, fostered and a sense of mystery that goes along with this whole documentary about *The Exorcist*. We're documenting something that is highly mysterious and to try to get it down in black and white so that people understand it thoroughly is impossible. That's why the empirical scientist just has to throw up his hands in despair and say, "I don't know anything about this, it doesn't occur so far as I'm concerned, and that's part of it." Well, I haven't really heard of that. I would say that it's extremely dangerous. Mock anything is dangerous, when we insist on saying that it's something else, we're doing a deliberate deception. Now in art, and television, and in the creative areas of life, that's understood and we all understood [interruption].

Can an exorcism really drive out an evil spirit?

O: There is a lot that would go under the rubric of driving out of evil spirits and that has a long, long history, not just limited to some Judeo-Christian tradition at all. The medicine man does that sort of thing. And a very good treatment of that within the psychiatric tradition was done by Jerome Frank several decades ago at around that time he was president of the American Psychiatric Association. And he wrote a whole book on the healing done by the shaman, the medicine man, the exorcist, the spiritual representative of the divinity in human cultures historically. It's a beautiful treatment. Obviously, the metaphorical usages, and some of them are purely metaphorical, and some of them are seriously meant, that there are diabolical spirits that dwell in us and must be driven out. But there's a terrible mixture in this eclecticism that is very hard to diagnose what they are talking about when they talk about driving out evil spirits. Some of it's, well, I'll tell you, some of it is quite analogous [fade out] to what my mother used to do when we kids were sick. She would put her hand on our forehead, and the mockery, or the simulation, if you will, was she was saying, "I'm going to feel your temperature." Do you have a temperature? That was a beautiful, beautiful act of comforting and help in sickness and it was one of the happiest memories I have of my childhood. Now that sort of thing ... the laying on of the hands, it was a lying on of hands. And that's a symbol that reflects not only the spirit, but also our humanity. Laying on hands is a human act that touches us.

What is the real evil in humans?

O: I think Father Halloran's statement is beautiful, because the evil in this world that we have to deal with, is, and this I mean deliberately, to refer that exorcism is not evil out there that impinges upon us, it's the evil in our hearts. And our job in life is to drive out that evil, the internal evil, the habitual evil, the evil we don't even recognize, and replace it with the gentle, loving, kindly philosophy of life that is interested in being there for other people. That was the summary motto of the former general of the Society of Jesus, the Jesuit general, Men for Others, and that's life, and that's why Father Halloran's comment is marvelous, yes, that's what the 21st century should be. Our preoccupation with our own problems of evil inside of us. How can I be a better human being with the human being I'm in contact with at this moment? Not is some extra-terrestrial spirit going to take over my life. The answer to that question is, no he's not! Get to work! Love a lot! And forget all this stuff about what's going to happen. Our role in that respect, with respect to that danger or evil, if to trust the dear Lord, and that's it. So. Yes, mostly by fighting evil here at home. Am I, was I mean today? Did I kick the car? Did I spout off at one of my students, or co-workers, or one of the cameramen or something like that?

In spite of evil in the world, will redemption from God come?

O: There's a ton of horrible stuff, and if you pursue that metaphor, there are a million and millions and millions of tons of good stuff. A Christian has to be optimistic, and I'm a Christian. So God's providence rules in the world, and he has redeemed the world, and the good guys—and in that respect Hollywood is right; it's one of the few things they are right about—in the long run, God does win out. We live in a redeemed world in the end period of human history, the final economy of salvation. And God is winning, has been winning, has been winning, is going to win. And the prophets of doom forget it. They're just silly. They don't have any faith, and they don't have any trust, and they haven't met the good providential God. And they're the ones who are in the most danger of making of the exorcism theme a melodramatic, sentimental ode to evil. Without knowing it.

Did the devil win in The Exorcist *movie?*

O: Oh, my goodness. That sort of exaggeration always undoes itself, and it's always destructive, and it has to be rebuilt within the providence of God. You might say that the unhappy ending of Blatty's first film plays right into that. But notice that the last chapter of his book, and the last scene in the film are not the last scenes of this whole scenario. For one thing, thank God that Discovery came along and did a serious documentary on this, and changed this whole view from a sentimental, silly, superficial view to something that is seriously historical, and seriously historical in the most important sense: In the economy of God's own providence and salvation for the human race. The devil never wins definitely, never, and that's the point I think, the ultimate point that has to be made by this documentary. Devils don't win. Good guys, and good guys in no superficial sense. We use the term in such a silly way, almost the same way we use love. No, God is the really good guy, and God is love, and love always wins. That's it, over and out.

Recollections from the First Exorcism: Father Frank Bobber

How did you meet Father Hughes?

Bobber: In 1980, the early part of that year, I transferred out to St. Raphael's in Potomac, Maryland, to St. James in Mount Rainier, and Fr. Hughes was the pastor at that point, and I became his associate pastor. From the beginning, we hit it off very well; many people though that we were a father and son team. We looked very much alike; in fact, my dad died when he was 57, and photographs of my dad were very similar to Fr. Hughes. So we hit off very well, we became good friends very quickly. Father Hughes was the type of an individual who loved lengthy dinner conversations. Primarily, we would have dinner probably beginning about 5:30 and it would go to around 7:30. You know, he liked just conversing, chatting, and enjoyed that because he was a very interesting person.

Where is Mount Rainier located?

B: Mount Rainier is a very historical old type of town, very familiar in a sense. Many families who, even to this day, live in Mt. Rainier have been there forever. For instance, many times when the dads and moms were to expire, you know, die, the children would take over their homes. So Mount Rainier is a very congenial area, very amicable, and as I say, very old, historically very significant for our state. In fact, it is my understanding that many years ago, before the advent of the air conditioning, senators of the White House, congresspeople would go to Mt. Rainier for the summer to escape the heat of DC itself. So it had a reputation.

Can you talk to us about his personality? Was he affected by the exorcism?

B: Well, I'd probably say there were two dimensions that I would focus on. The first dimension was prior to his doing the exorcism, a dimension that I was familiar with, because as I mentioned, I had gone there in 1980. In this earlier dimension, from my understanding from a lot of parishioners, who I said had lived there forever and know Father Hughes very well, said he was an extremely amiable, gregarious type of individual. He had served both as an associate pastor and in due time as a pastor. Now, as I say, prior to the exorcism he was a fun, full type of an individual and very gregarious. Subsequent to the exorcism, and this is of course when I came to know him in due time, he was far more of an introvert than before; he was an extrovert earlier. He became an introvert, a person who was very much a person of prayer, a person who very much kept to himself. Also, my dinners with him, the conversations, from what I understood, were rare. You know, normally he did not care to spend much time with anyone. But we did hit it off, but there was that incredible transition from an extrovert to an introvert. From a gregarious type of a person [to one] who preferred being by himself.

Did you know he was the pastor involved in the initial part of the Mount Rainier Exorcism?

B: OK, when I received directions form the Archdiocese that I was going to be transferred from St. Raphael's in Potomac, Maryland, to Mount Rainier St. James, several people approached me, once the news became public. They said, do you realize where you are going and whom you are going with? I answered yes, and I am like, well, Mt. Rainier, I had no idea of Mt. Rainier's significance. And they asked me if I had seen the movie *The Exorcist* and I said, well, yes. Then they mentioned to me that he was the priest that was initially involved with the exorcism that became the primary focus for the film *The Exorcist*. And I was like, wow, so I was so excited. I thought this could be a new dimension for my life. But at that point in time I was not sure of the veracity of this; only in terms of the facts. Often times one hears rumors and things of that nature. But when I did go to St. James, one evening I mustered up the courage and I was having dinner with Father Hughes and we were alone and I said, "Father Al, I heard that you were the priest that was involved in the story, the exorcism that became part of the film *The Exorcist*. Is that true?" So he looked at me and said that is true.

Did he provide you with more information?

B: No, at that point is all that all he told me was that he was involved. He did not say too much that evening, but one reason probably because when I mustered up the courage to present this question, we had already been at the table like two hours. So there were appointments and so soon, we both of us agreed to approach this subject at our next dinner conversation, which was the case.

Did you have the next dinner together?

B: It was most interesting. It was a very lengthy conversation and I had numerous questions, and for some strange reason he was very open with me. He did mention that he was not all that open, discussing the things about the exorcism primarily of the memory associated with it. It was very painful, but, ah, because of our relationship he was willing to pursue it. As I said, I had many questions and he was very responsive. He told how it began, the process....

What did he tell you about the process?

B: Originally, if my memory serves me correctly, it was a Lutheran minister, the mom and dad of the youngster were Lutherans and they had gone to see their minister, a Lutheran minister, in terms of this extraordinary experience their son was going through that apparently psychologists and medical people could not fathom. And they went to see their minister and their minister told them that the Roman Catholic Church does deal with possession and exorcism and things of that nature. So he had suggested just go up the street to the Catholic Church, St. James, Father Hughes was associate there, and see a priest and discuss it with him, and that is what happened.

What is the story?

B: What they said to him was that their son was—and I think he was 12 or 13 years old at the time—he was experiencing extremely bizarre phenomena.

You know, that they had taken him for medical analysis, medical treatment and the doctors were basically beside themselves. They were not really making any headway with him, and they were very perplexed about the entire situation. So, they were informed I guess through a friend that, or maybe one of the doctors, that this maybe had to do with more than a medical problem. It could have been more of a spiritual problem. He brought the boy over to the rectory. Fr. Hughes at that point, after talking with mom and dad and the boy and witnessing certain elements, he thought that it would be appropriate to contact the archbishop at that time to see if this case may warrant an exorcism. He said there were very strange phenomena. He mentioned that in his office where he met with the boy and the mom and dad that the boy was able to look at the phone and move the phone across the room. The boy was not happy at all being there interviewed by the priest, and he articulated this in very foul language and whatnot. And Fr. Hughes told me that the room got very cold, you know, frigid. So he said that those things themselves were a bit scary. Ah, he spoke at a level that was far more basic than a 12- or 13-year-old boy kind of like an adult. Very rudimentary. That's what Hughes told me.

Was Hughes terrified?

B: Yes, yes, he was. Because Fr. Hughes at that point in time was young, ordained just a few years. As often with most priests, after you finish the seminary, [you] may be more prone to scientific interpretations of things. Exorcism is not popular today as it was many years ago. During the medieval ages, it was very common; today it is not. Today the Church, though the Church recognizes that possession may certainly occur, in most situations where there is a possibility, the Church prefers that the person would be studied medically, etc., and that hopefully there would be some type of medical response to the situation. You know, epilepsy or whatever. So the Church is not all that comfortable with it. But there are times when medical science says this is beyond our domain, and then the Church will get involved.

Once Father Hughes determined that it was a case of demonic possession, did he ask the Church for permission to perform the exorcism?

B: And then Fr. Hughes approached the archdioceses, because in the Catholic Church to validly perform an exorcism you need to get the permission from the archbishop or the bishop. So he approached—at that time it was Archbishop O'Boyle, and I don't think Father Hughes was that interested in doing it himself, but he just gave the case to the archbishop. But then Archbishop O'Boyle asked him to do it, so that was the beginning of the process.

Did he consult the Roman Ritual for this case?

B: Yes, he read up on it. There is a Ritual in Roman Catholicism that lists, for example, blessings of numerous objects, certain types of prayers; it includes also the rite for exorcism. So he did that. He read up on it, as is customary before a priest gets involved in exorcism, you fast, you pray a lot, which he did. So he prepared himself in that sense. Then the parents brought the boy back and he began the ritual. The rite itself [was performed at] the rectory, then in the boy's home and then eventually at Georgetown Hospital because the boy was getting progressively more violent.

How did Father Hughes get injured during the exorcism?

B: The hospital situation was very climactic; Fr. Hughes told me that the boy was for the exorcism process, they had him strapped down on the bed. At one point, Fr. Hughes said that he was going through the wordings of the rite and the boy snapped with his right hand the strap and went underneath the bed and grabbed one of the hospital springs—you know, bed springs—and pulled it out and slashed Fr. Hughes's arm. It was his left arm. And of course, he went into screaming and hollering, Fr. Hughes that is, and nurses rushed in and he needed medical attention. He showed me the scar too, which was interesting. And at that point he said he cannot handle this any longer, it is too draining on his part, and that's when the Jesuits became involved. They took the boy to St. Louis, Missouri, to a hospital that is run by the Alexian Brothers, and two Jesuit priests pursued the exorcism, the rites thereof which eventually worked out.

Did this exorcism of Ronald fail?

B: He never said why he did not think, it did not work. I would surmise it was based on the idea that he was newly ordained, he was a neophyte in this area and normally ... the priests who do exorcisms are usually well-trained, they are missionary priests often. They are people who are very familiar with the rites, and as I say, Fr. Hughes was very young, he was an associate pastor. So, for him, I think he believed that he was just not strong enough theologically or spiritually to deal with this.

Did he believe that he dealt with the real Devil?

B: Ah ... as I say, ultimately the exorcism was successful, so Satan was not, in that sense, but in this process, I think Fr. Hughes felt he was no match for dealing with Satan.

He really feels he was dealing with Satan?

B: Oh, yes. In fact, I remember one evening we were having a discussion, and he mentioned, he said, "You know, Frank, often times you do think that things like Satan, possessions, exorcism are not realities, they are some things that are relegated to the superstitious." And he said, "I for a long time thought that this was something that was in that realm, too, until I came to deal with the devils in this kid's case." And he said he just changed his mind totally, he said he became a very strong believer. In fact, that conversation I remember,

I said to him, most of us young priests, because I was just ordained myself at that point, we're in that same boat. We are not so sure what is myth and what is fact. Reality. Why don't you give us a seminar and just inform the priests in the archdiocese, the younger priests? Do it primarily for the young priests, who are interested in it and just inform them of your experiences.

Did he decide to help younger priests to understand demonic possession and exorcism?

B: He agreed to it, he agreed to it, but then the following week he died, had a massive heart attack. I think this dinner, in which I had mentioned this to him, was a Friday, and on Sunday he celebrated mass, and after mass he left to [go to] Baltimore to [visit] some relatives. And Monday night there was a parish council meeting and he didn't show, which was unusual. I was a bit concerned, but I thought he just got tied up with something. And then about midnight, the police called me to tell me they found him dead.

What happened to him after the exorcism?

B: In fact, several people from Mt. Rainier, who had lived there for years and had known Fr. Hughes as an associate pastor and pastor, did mention and in fact they even gave [statements] to the news media, ah, newspaper reporters. It is important to note that prior to the exorcism he was an extremely handsome young man, black hair, curly. Subsequent to the exorcism, his hair was white; he looked as if he had aged incredibly. So they had talked about some very radical physical transformations.

If he was young and a newcomer to the priesthood, why did he accept to perform the exorcism?

B: Well, I think that he never really got into why he thought he could … most priests, [when] you are first ordained, you're zealous, you're enthusiastic. You are ready to take on the world for Jesus. And I'm sure when the archbishop said to him, "I want you to do it," he probably said, "Well, OK, I will." He was young enough, enthusiastic, zealous, and thought, well, this will be a big challenge, but I'm up for it.

Was this experience very traumatic for him?

B: From my conversations with him, I think he would not have ventured into that. He would have told the archbishop get someone else to do it, if he knew what was going to happen. Because that exorcism, it was very traumatic for him. The Church, generally speaking, is very private, secretive, quiet when it comes [to] things like exorcism, for a number of reasons. One reason, of course, is to maintain the identity of the individual involved. Ah … keep that secret. Secondly, the Church, knowing those years ago that people who suffered from epilepsy, or psychotic problems, often times were labeled as being possessed. And the Church does not want to associate herself with that type of a situation. So, the Church tends to be very private and quiet about these kinds of things. Recognizing at the same time that it does happen, but there are cases that are reported to be cases of possession that turn out to be just psychotic situations ... illnesses.

Did the media ever approach you on the Mount Rainier case?

B: I think it was in 1983, the *Washington Post* came to see me ... well, not the *Post* but the ... the newspeople from the *Post* when I was at St. Stephen's. They wanted to do sort of a research study of Mt. Rainier, because they were informed of incredible numbers of bizarre evil criminal actions or elements. Ah ... for example, not far from the house where the boy and the parents lived, police found a woman in a plastic bag, her body decomposing. A couple doors away from that house, a guy went crazy and decapitated his mother. Um, a few doors down from those, children were arrested for hacking off appendages of their parents. So that entire area there seemed to be plagued by very bizarre criminal elements. In fact, I remember when the *Post* did an article on this, I received a letter from a young man who was serving a life sentence up in Jessup, Maryland. And he told me, he said that he, you know, was convicted of having hacked his mother to death. You know, several pieces. It was awful and he told me, in the letter, "I am not asking for leniency or intervention. I just wanted you to know some power possessed me." That is what he said and I still have that letter to date. Ah, and he says, you know, "Please don't go to the courts on my behalf. I just wanted you to know that there is something extraordinarily uncomfortable about Mt. Rainier." That is what he said. "I did this and I loved my mom, but," he said, "some power just took over me and I hacked her to pieces." And then of course was arrested and is serving a life sentence now.

How does evil work through a person?

B: I am not so certain as to how the powers of evil work. If specifically, through a person or if a locus becomes a situation, I don't know. But sometimes if you think about somebody like Adolf Hitler, for example, you have a person who was very comfortable with the physical extermination of 6 million Jews, one million of which were children, and many of them died in a very barbaric fashion, laboratory experiments, and whatnot. How do you answer that? How can a human being do that, and still be considered a human being? And if a locus, a location can be privative to strange phenomena, well, maybe, I don't know.

Do you and Fr. Hughes believe this was truly a case of demonic possession?

B: Yes, he certainly did, and I do too, after he related his experiences with the boy, all these things, speaking in ancient languages, superhuman strength, the incredible discomfort with holy, sacred things. He certainly came to the conclusion that is satanic possession. And although I had not had that experience, I've always thought of Fr. Hughes as being a bright person with lots of integrity, honesty. So, there was no reason for me to think that he was lying, and besides that, I have been in much contact with Fr. Nicola, who is like the world's primary demonologist.

Did the boy speak in a different language?

B: Yes, Fr. Hughes was not able to discern what the languages were. But the boy was subject to psychiatric analysis, and they did determine when they recorded some of his saying and they had that subject to linguistic analysis, he would be speaking, like, ancient Greek, Aramaic. You know … languages that are not alive, you know. Popular today, yes, he would hear the boy speaking. But you know, as I say, it was, specifically, when the team of psychiatrists and psychologists studied the boy.

Did he witness any marks being produced by the Devil in the adolescent's body?

B: He said on his chest there were all kinds of cryptic markings that would appear during the rites of exorcism. I use the term cryptic because Fr. Hughes could not translate those markings themselves.

He never thought the boy was faking or a hoax?

B: No, he was 100 percent positive that this was way beyond the boy's capacity. You know, even the strength to break a strap, hospital strap, to pull out, you know, a coil from under the bed was superhuman.

Do you think a 13-year-old normal adolescent would not be able to do that?

B: Yeah, a 13-year-old could never do that. Even an adult probably could not do that. So it was a very unusual experience for him. And he believed. As he told me, he said prior to then he maybe would have not questioned the existence of Satan, but he certainly would have questioned possession or obsession, as they say in technical terms. But subsequent to that experience, he had no questions of it happening.

Did this experience deepen his faith?

B: It deepened, it deepened his faith considerably. In fact, he became extremely faithful to God. Or I should say a person of extreme prayer, subsequent to [the exorcism]. He believed, he told me, he came very much to believe in the power of the priesthood.

Was he convinced that he was dealing with the unknown?

B: Well, I think what we can possibly learn is that we are all faced with the unknown and we have to struggle to cope with the unknown and perhaps the best element in struggling to cope with the unknown is a deep faith in God. If you really believe that there is a God and you really believe that God is involved in human life and God is a loving, caring parent, that faith can help to you cope with whatever happens. Today they talk about finding artifacts that indicate former life on Mars. Maybe someday we will be involved with life from other planets, intelligent life. It possibly may not be very benign, but once again, if one believes in a loving, caring God, that faith will help one to cope successfully with whatever situation arises.

The Sacred, Psychic and Science: Dr. Sergio A. Rueda, Ph.D.

Dr. Sergio Antonio Rueda, author of this book, is a specialist in behavioral medicine at the Institute of Medicine and Advanced Behavioral Technologies in El Paso, Texas. He is also a trained theologian and expert in biblical languages.

How did you learn about the Mount Rainier Exorcism and its relation to
The Exorcist?
Rueda: Well, while I was a visiting scholar at the Institute of Parapsychology in Durham, North Carolina, I found some documents that were related to the case, the Mount Rainier case, such as the correspondence between J.B. Rhine and the Reverend Father Luther Miles Schulze regarding the case on which the film *The Exorcist* had been based.

Why did you decide to investigate the case?
R: At the Institute for Parapsychology, I had obtained a grant from the Parapsychology Foundation of New York to investigate the Mount Rainier case. I had found at the Institute for Parapsychology in Durham, North Carolina, some letters related to the case, which I had found in the archives of the institute, and that is how I got interested in the Mount Rainier Case and *The Exorcist.* I then made a research proposal on the case to the Parapsychology Foundation of New York and I obtained a research grant to investigate it. They knew about the relevance of the case for researchers and the general public and decided to support my proposal. As far as I know, this was the first time in the history of research in anomalistic phenomena that a grant had been granted to investigate this case from a scientific standpoint.

What was the Reverend Schulze's explanation of this case in his letters to J.B. Rhine?
R: Basically, the Reverend Schulze's explanation to Dr. J.B. Rhine was that he was facing an apparent case of poltergeist activity in which paranormal phenomena was apparently involved.

Well, what was your hypothesis about the causality of these phenomena?
R: Well, any good scientist must first have to consider the case "in the context of science," and the first hypothesis that came to mind was a medical

hypothesis. I asked myself, is there a medical explanation for the phenomena reported in the case? I also got interested from the perspective of the parapsychological phenomena, as a possible explanation for the phenomena that took place in the Mount Rainier case. I approached the case from a scientific standpoint initially. I considered the entire possible explanatory hypothesis, such as psychological, medical, fraud, and even tried to assess the demonic possession agency hypothesis.

In my opinion, when we approach a phenomenon of a paranormal nature such as the one reported in the Mount Rainier case, we first need to approach the case with a scientific methodology and consider also the possibility of fraud, since it has been found in the history of the investigation of paranormal phenomena that many cases have been found the result of clever trickery. For instance, in one of the most famous cases in the paranormal literature, such as the Columbus Poltergeist, the alleged subject of the paranormal activity was found doing tricks.

In the Mount Rainier Exorcism, it seems to me rather suspicious that the boy showed some marks on this body that appeared, apparently, spontaneously. Interestingly, most of the time he was out of the view of his family members during the initial stage of the case, so the apparent spontaneous marks appear on his body but no one saw them appear spontaneously. Also, there is another element of the case that made me suspect that fraud may have taken place. The reason being, for this fraud, that the boy had a motive to cause the marks himself to avoid going to school, where he was having problems with classmates, so that he would be allowed to go to live with his preferred aunt in St. Louis. For instance, he wanted to go to live in St. Louis with his preferred aunt, a desire that emerges at the same time that he was having difficulties at school. Therefore, he may have inflicted the marks on himself in order to avoid going to school. I have the impression that the 14-year-old adolescent may have manufactured some of the marks to scare his family and accomplish his motive to avoid an unpleasant stimulus.

What happened to the adolescent's aunt?

R: Oh, she died. Interestingly, when she died the phenomena stopped. Probably the boy got discouraged and he decided to stop the ordeal. Moreover, the family was very superstitious. Instead of seeking out medical help for the boy, they instead sought the help of a spiritualist to rid the boy of the problem by doing some form of spiritual anointing. This ritual is called the Powai. By the way, the Reverend Schulze was present when the person arrived to perform the Powai ritual. Also the family was upset because of the Reverend Schulze's skeptical attitude. So the Powai person arrived and she performed some sort of magic tricks to prove she had some kind of powers, and the Reverend Schulze confronted her and he replicated the tricks that she performed to demonstrate that she had no powers. So the spiritualist person thought that the Reverend Schulze had stolen some of her thunder, so she was pretty upset about it, but the family was annoyed with Schulze's attitude and decided to take him out of the case.

Did the family belong to any religious group?
    R: Yes, they were members of the Reverend Schulze's St. Stephen's Lutheran Church, and they decided to seek out first the assistance of their personal minister. That's why they contacted him first. Initially, they told him that something strange was happening at home, and that they believed that the Devil was trying to interfere with their family and perhaps their son was possessed by the Devil.

And what did the Reverend Schulze do?
    R: Actually, he took a very skeptical and guarded position. He first considered that perhaps the boy was playing some tricks to deceive the family. Also that the adolescent himself was trying to convey a message to the mother so that she would let him go to St. Louis to live with his preferred aunt. For instance, the mother was very interested in Spiritualism and spirit communication, and the adolescent took advantage of this and he tried to convey the message via some clever tricks so that the family would let him go to St. Louis.

But what did Schulze see?
    R: Well, first he asked the family to allow the adolescent to stay at his parsonage for one night to find out by himself if the boy was manufacturing some tricks or was it a genuine phenomenon. He took the adolescent to his parsonage, but he was shaken by what he witnessed. He witnessed phenomena that initially he thought were being caused by some clever tricks by the adolescent. For instance, he reported that during the night the adolescent spent at his house, he placed the boy in the bed before going to sleep but he was shaken by what happened next. The bed vibrated when he placed him on it. He repeated the placing of the adolescent in the bed to find out if the phenomenon would repeat. However, whenever he put the boy in the bed, the bed would begin to shake. Surprised by this, then he decided to place the adolescent on a blanket on the floor, but then to his surprise, the blanket began to glide with the boy on it under the bed. Also at one point, the bed threw him out of it. Regarding his attitude about witnessing this phenomenon taking place in front of him, the Reverend Schulze declared that he maintained a very close observation of the phenomena with the hypothesis in mind that the adolescent was playing very smart tricks to create such phenomena. He was still very much skeptical about the phenomena he witnessed. Still, the hands of the adolescent and body were standing still as the phenomena

took place, and as well, he did not see his hands moving. Therefore, that night he was surprised about what he witnessed.

How did the boy make the bed shake?

R: The Reverend Schulze told me that he did not have an explanation for that; in my opinion, this phenomenon is perhaps the strongest evidence in favor of the poltergeist hypothesis for this case. An explanation for that phenomenon is that, somehow, energy inside of the adolescent gets transferred outside as energy causing the movement of objects, which may be of a poltergeist nature, as some experts in the field of anomalistic psychology claim.

How about the bed shaking and the bed made on the floor that glided under the bed?

R: Personally, I cannot account for this phenomenon, but I believe this may be some case of poltergeist phenomenon. It is typical that this phenomenon takes place in this kind of case. Furniture moves around, strange sounds are heard; marks may appear on the body of the poltergeist subject. A lot of that stuff is reported in some poltergeist cases investigated by experts in the field of anomalistic psychology.

How heavy was the chair where the adolescent was sat down by the Reverend Schulze? It is reported that the adolescent sat in a heavy chair and that it moved without any movement made by the adolescent.

R: The Reverend Schulze, told me, it was a low-gravity chair, that it was quite heavy and it moved about 7 inches and it then hit the wall and it flipped over.

How did the Reverend Schulze explain this phenomenon?

R: According to him, he was never able to explain these phenomena at all. He considered that it may have been the result of a poltergeist phenomenon. He explained to me that, because he had read some of the books by J.B. Rhine regarding paranormal phenomena, he had considered that the pattern of this case was similar to that observed in poltergeist activity.

Was he a parapsychologist?

R: No, he was a Lutheran minster, but he was familiar with the parapsychological literature.

Did he try to find a solution for the case?

R: Evidently, he was shaken by the phenomena he had witnessed and tried to find medical expertise to explain it. Also, he was familiar with the work on parapsychology conducted by J.B. Rhine at Duke University Parapsychology Laboratory, and decided to contact him to see if he could help him out finding a suitable explanation for the phenomena. He wrote to J.B.

Rhine, who is considered the father of modern parapsychology; they started a mutual correspondence where Dr. Rhine tried to guide Schulze to determine the nature of the phenomena. Moreover, in response to his letter asking for help, Dr. J.B. Rhine asks him to take a guarded position, also to be skeptical about the phenomenon. The reason being that, according to Dr. J.B. Rhine, there have been cases in the history of poltergeist-like phenomena that had been found to be fake and in which trickery had been detected, particularly when the phenomena surrounded a young adolescent. In this particular case, we have an adolescent who was undergoing some serious psychological deep-seated stress or conflict.

Do you yourself believe in demonic possession?
    R: I think, before we discuss demonic possession, we first need to discuss whether or not the Devil does exist. The existence of demonic possession, in my opinion, is conditioned on the existence of the Devil, and there is no way we can prove the existence of the devil in an indisputable manner. This is a church dogma that we believe by faith and believe it for this case in the context of the Catholic Church.

How would you explain the Mount Rainier Case?
    R: Personally, it would be hard to explain the case by singling out just one cause. I think, since a long time ago, researchers on anomalistic psychology realized that poltergeist-like phenomena are not completely genuine nor completely fake or phony. So there must be some element, some pattern to determine real, genuine poltergeist-like cases. What we know is that in most of the cases, where an adolescent is involved, trickery has been detected. Consequently, in my personal view, fraud may have been involved in this at least at the initial stages of the ordeal. Moreover, after carefully studying the case, as an expert in mental health, I believe that the child was suffering from a psychological conflict that became a disorder known as conversion reaction, in which a person has a psychological motive to avoid a noxious stimulus. Therefore, mental somatizations are present, unconsciously, which helps the person avoid the negative stimulus we no longer want to face. For instance, a soldier does not want to go to war and, suddenly, one of his arms gets paralyzed. Ah, furthermore, I believe the case may have been of a poltergeist nature and was converted into a demonic possession case by the decision to exorcise the boy. As an expert on demonic possession once said, "If you call the devil you will see the devil." And if you do not see the Devil, you will see the manifestations of person's ideas of it. So it is my impression, based on my research and all the details of the case, that a case that had begun as obsession and a poltergeist case, was converted into possession by the decision of the priest to perform the exorcism.

What was the family's approach to solve the case?

R: The family made the decision to proceed with an exorcism, after the Reverend Schulze suggested that the Catholics were interested in the topic and perhaps they might have some way of helping the child. That is how they began to contact the Catholic Church. However, the Reverend Schulze continued to be interested in the case and also gathered information and continued the correspondence on the case with Dr. J.B. Rhine in order to find out what was the real cause of the phenomena. Nevertheless, he took a very scientific position; he also tried to investigate the case from a medical standpoint. First, he suggested medical treatment to the family; he suggested that the boy be put in the hands of a medical doctor that would be sympathetic to the adolescent. Secondly, he tried to find out if trickery was the cause of the phenomenon. Thirdly, he investigated the poltergeist phenomena surrounding the boy, so he went through all the steps to find out if there was a natural cause in order to rule out all those aspects.

What did the family do?

R: They followed to some extent what the Reverend Schulze suggested; however, they didn't like that idea very much to take the adolescent to medical treatment. At some point, they got very annoyed and they declined the participation of Schulze and his doctor in the case. They were superstitious and decided to seek the help of a spiritualist who would perform the Powai ritual on the adolescent. The Powai is some sort of ritual in which evil spirits are exorcised by some sort of confirmations and things like that. The Reverend Schulze was present when the Powai doctor arrived to perform the ritual at the house of the Hunkelers. Interestingly, the Powai person tried to show the Reverend Schulze that she had some powers. Also, that she had the right to be there to cure the boy because she had the actual knowledge to do it. Next, the Powai doctor decided to show a magic trick to show she had some powers. In response to this, the Reverend Schulze replicated the trick and said, "Look I can do the same thing, you don't have any powers." Finally, the Reverend Schulze left the house a little bit upset by what the family was doing with the case.

Did you know Father Hughes?

R: With Fr. Hughes, I do not know much about his participation, but it seems like a family friend of them, recommended him to assist the family with the case. So he was the first priest, but I don't think Hughes was involved in that decision.

Once the Catholics got involved, what happened?

R: Unfortunately, they took a very light position on the case, they evaluated the case very fast and they made a quick decision to perform an exorcism in only five days.

Who made the decision to perform the exorcism?

R: Father Bowdern and Father Halloran both went to the family's house on March the 10th, 1949, and on the 11th, while they were in the house, there were some phenomena that took place that was in Mt. Rainier. So while they were there and the family was providing them with an update on the case, what was going on, and also they were getting the details of the case. At one point of the conversation, Father Halloran decided to place a religious relic on the boy's pillow and then he came downstairs and continued talking to the family. Next, while he was talking to the family, they heard Ronald yelling, and both Father Bowdern and Halloran dashed up along with the family to see what was happening, and when they asked Ronald about the reason of the yelling, Ronald told them that a crucifix or whatever religious relic that was there rose from the pillow and struck a mirror, but they did not witness the phenomenon. Once the boy calmed down and relaxed, they went downstairs and continued to discuss the issue. Again, while they were discussing the issue, again something else happened. A bottle of holy water that had placed on a table landed six feet from the table. The same story: Ronald yelled for help, the priests dashed up again to see what had happened, he reported to them what had happened in that event, but they did not witness any of the phenomena.

The next day or the following days, they took, Bowdern and Halloran, some kind of crash course in demonic possession; they read some theological works on obsession, which is what they taught was taking place in the case of Ronald. In the following days, after having studied the case in the context of the Roman Rituale, they got the approval to perform an exorcism and proceeded to perform it with the family's permission.

Next, let's talk about parapsychology, which is one of the explanations to account for the phenomena in this case.

R: Parapsychology is the study of paranormal phenomena or ESP, in other words, you can gather information or you can obtain information from the environment without your senses mediating it. In other words, you can acquire knowledge from an external source without using your normal five senses. In some way, you know, you can connect with some information either in the future or at a distance. For instance, like if someone con read someone else's mind or become aware of your internal thinking processes.

What is the Reverend Schulzes attitude toward the case after so many years?

R: Interestingly, so many years after the original case took place, he was still so much of a skeptic about the phenomena. He still believed that something was happening there, but it was not a demon that was causing it. He didn't believe that Ronald was possessed at all; he was more inclined to believe that some sort of strange forces, possibly, like poltergeist forces were acting in the case. Poltergeist forces are a phenomenology that is manifested particularly when a child is undergoing a psychological conflict, deep-seated stress. Some experts on anomalistic psychology believed that inner stress gets externalized through those manifestations. Usually the victim of this phenomenon is undergoing psychological stress, which for some experts is connected to the developing sexual energies. So it is believed that this phenomenon is a result of that conflict.

How is demonic possession diagnosed?

R: There is no official procedure to diagnose it from a psychological or psychiatric standpoint. However, by the Catholic Church, which in order to establish that demonic possession exists in a particular person or that a person is possessed by the Devil, they have certain rules. The Catholic Church has established some criteria in the Roman Ritual published in 1614 at the request of a Pope. In these criteria, we find that there are some symptoms which are considered to be indicative of possession. Among them, if the person is able to speak in a foreign language which the possessed has not learned previously. Secondly, if the person has knowledge of hidden things about events and persons without having had previous access to this information at all from any other natural source. Thirdly, if the person possessed shows superhuman strength. However, we don't see any of those symptoms in the particular case of Ronald; consequently, in the context of the signs of possession indicated in the Roman Ritual, the case does not meet the requirement to be diagnosed as such.

Then why did they diagnose it as such by the Catholic priests?

R: I think Father Bowdern and Father Halloran considered that the next step in obsession was going to be possession, and therefore in order to avoid possession, they thought that it was a good idea to stop it there when it was still obsession. In obsession, the Devil focuses his powers on the person and afflicts the person either psychologically or physically, but it doesn't reach the stage of possession. For instance, the person may suffer scratches on the body; also the Devil may attack the person one way or another, but it doesn't reach the level of possession. In possession, the stage of full possession of the individual by the Devil takes place.

What are the stages of demonic possession?

R: The first stage is called "infestation." In infestation some strange sounds may be produced in the house. Some strange phenomena take place where people can't really account for it, how this phenomenon is produced. So that is the process of infestation: it is like poltergeist phenomena or activity that suggest the possibility of a diabolical presence. The second stage is called obsession. Once infestation takes place and the Devil becomes more active, it begins to attack the person in a personal way, so the Devil might attack the person via physical attacks or the person might get hit with furniture or things like that. Then, the next step would be possession, so Halloran and Bowdern considered that the next step in the case was going to be possession. So by proceeding with exorcism they would avoid the possession stage or stop it.

How about the marks that appeared on the boy's body? How would you explain them?

R: Well, if the marks truly appeared. There is some evidence in the letters from Schulze addressed to J.B. Rhine about these marks, and he mentioned that he saw some of the marks. However, the Reverend Schulze explained that he didn't see clear marks; for him they there were like some nerve rashes that look like scratches. Those marks, interestingly, contained messages against going to school; in other words, the boy didn't want to go to school. It is important to note that he was having a difficult time in school, such as having some difficulties interacting with other students. Therefore, in order to avoid the problems he was having in school, he decided to stop going. In my opinion, there was a motive on the part of the boy to avoid attending school. First, he wanted to go to live with his preferred aunt, who lived in St. Louis, Missouri. So I consider that the boy was trying to convey a message to his mother that in some way, the spirits wanted him to go to St. Louis. So in my opinion, it is quite likely that he was making the marks on himself to convey the mysterious message. Furthermore, that he was suffering from a psychological condition known as "conversion reaction." In conversion reaction, psychic energies get converted into the body symptoms and when the person suffers from the condition, he or she is trying generally to avoid a noxious stimulus. In this particular case, Ronald was trying to avoid going to school because he was having some difficulties there. However, he was suffering from an actual psychological condition like conversion reaction, in which the skin becomes so sensitive that if you use just your fingernails and move them over the surface of the skin, you may create marks on your body. This is because the skin is so sensitive, so I think that when he was out of the view of the family, that condition helped him make the marks on himself.

Furthermore, he could have made them on his own body, perhaps, by scratching up against the wall for the marks that were not easy to be made on his body. Interestingly, most of the marks indicate that he did not want to go to school. For instance, two big "N"s appeared on both of his legs and the word "N" indicating "NO" appeared on his wrists. When they were discussing the possibility for him to attend school while they were in St. Louis, his marks even denied such a possibility. Why would a spirit be so concerned for such futile details such as not attending school?

Did the Reverend Schulze see some words on the body of the adolescent?

R: Reverend Schulze told me that he didn't see the words such as St. Louis on the boy's body; he just said he saw some sort of skin rashes that looked like scratches. I believe the boy may have made the marks on himself, that some of them, if not all, maybe were manufactured by him. Also, in order to accomplish his goal to avoid going to school where he was having some problems. And also to go to live with his preferred aunt. These symptoms fit the DSM-IV criteria for conversion reaction. The person is trying to avoid the noxious stimulus and he gains something out of it, so he chooses the symptoms that can allow him/her to obtain what is needed.

Was the family superstitious?

R: The family was rather superstitious. For instance, at one point they practiced a spiritualist séance in order to try to rid the adolescent from demonic possession.

Did the father and mother get along very well?

R: Yes, I have been informed they got along pretty well, except for something that was causing a problem in their relationship; for instance, that the father didn't have the command in making the decisions. The mother had the final word on making the family decision and the decisions on Ronald. Therefore, they had a conflict, for instance, on who would decide the kind education they wanted for Ronald. On the other hand, the mother wanted to send him to school no matter what problems he was having, such as the problems with the marks and the psychological condition. On the contrary, the father supported Ronald, he was a spoiled child for him; therefore, there was a conflict between the mother and the father. She wanted to send him to school, and he didn't want to send the boy to school. He was an only child.

Did you interview any friends close to the family?

R: Yes, I talked to several people who participated in the circle of prayers that was organized on behalf of the boy by members of his church.

What did they think about this case?

R: Most people had the tendency to exaggerate things. Some of them got information through gossip. Once the information breaks up to the general public, they began to exaggerate things. A lot of people believed it was a genuine phenomenon, some of them believed that they were faking it.

How was the relationship with their community?

R: I think they had a pretty good relationship with the community and, by the way, there was someone who participated in the circle of prayers who told me that while they were organizing the prayers at the home of the adolescent, they witnessed incredible phenomena, such as the bed rising from the floor, and it levitated and the boy was lying on the bed while they were praying.

Who did they think was causing these phenomena?
R: They attributed everything to the Devil. They were firm believers in the demonic possession agency. Ahh, a lot of people believed it was the Devil.

What did Schulze think about this situation?
R: Reverend Schulze felt they weren't being very scientific, particularly the priests. He was familiar with the Roman Ritual and the symptoms of possession [even though] he was a Lutheran minister, and he considered they were not being very scientific in their approach. Furthermore, I think he considered that the case was not being handled in the proper way because they were being so eager to accept all the facts that the family reported to them as truthful. So they took the testimonials that were reported to them as truthful and as if it they had really taken place. So I think the Reverend Schulze feeling was that the case was not being handled properly.

Do you believe this was a poltergeist case?
R: I think the case resembles those reported by parapsychologists in the literature related to poltergeist phenomena. I believe a case that began as a poltergeist case or infestation was converted into possession because of the decision to perform on exorcism. The adolescent didn't show the conventional signs of a demonic possession. In other words, they didn't have a case in favor of demonic possession. Still they proceeded to get the approval to perform the exorcism; I think that was an irresponsible decision on the part of the priests.

Why do you believe that?
R: Well, if you call the Devil, you may see the Devil, or rather, the victim's idea of the Devil. In other words, if [a person] can be induced to believe [he is possessed, he] can begin expressing [him]self like if [he] were possessed. Also, because you know the exorcism ritual is a very impressive ritual and may let yourself follow with the idea that it can free you from possession. People can be induced into believing that they are possessed and therefore they can begin acting out in that way.

Do you think somebody who is induced to believe that he/she is possessed can begin acting accordingly?
R: Exactly, if you were possessed, in addition to that, all the events that took place, all the phenomena that took place, and in spite of that, I don't see very strong evidence in favor that the adolescent was possessed. Also, [there were] all the events that were reported by the family, such as the shaking of a mattress and some marks, but as I said before, in some cases of conversion

reaction, people under a lot of stress can suffer from dermography and marks can easily appear. Also, a lot people heard him speaking in a loud voice and then he would reduce the pitch. Things and phenomena like that. But that doesn't seem to be something extraordinary to be taken as a sign of possession. The Roman Ritual indicates that the person has to be able to speak in a foreign language, and he didn't speak in a foreign language. The family reported to the Reverend Schulze that the boy spoke in a foreign language, but the Reverend Schulze said he never heard him speaking in a foreign language. So all we see is the exorcism at the Alexian Brothers Hospital, where the most extraordinary phenomena took place, such as the shaking of the mattress that, in my opinion, may be of a poltergeist nature, and the marks that may be explained by conversion reaction in which marks erupt. There may be a reddening of the skin when the person is under a lot of stress. Somehow, explain some experts on paranormal phenomena, the stress energy gets externalized by some unknown mechanism and causes the dermatological reactions. In other words, there may be a psychogenic origin for the marks.

Why do you think up to the present time people are interested in The Exorcist?

R: It has been so long since the book and film were originally released. I believe people are still interested because of the powerful influence of the film on moviegoers. No such dramatic events of the fight between good versus evil had been ever seen in any movie in such dramatized manner. I think the film created a collective psychosis of terror and absolutely, the film *The Exorcist* brought with it a lot of interest in this topic of demonic possession and exorcism that we had not seen before the movie. Even after 50 years that have passed, people still continue to be interested, because they always wonder about the events surrounding the origin of *The Exorcist*. What really happened? What was behind the film? Also, since the initial release of the movie, there were rumors that the film was based on an actual case, and that even increased the interest in the film. We must remember that the case, the Mount Rainier case on which the film was based, was recreated to make it appear as a real case of demonic possession. So that in the film, the case meets the requirements of the Roman Ritual, but the actual case was much less dramatic. In my opinion, the Mount Rainier case does not meet the requirements of the Roman Ritual to diagnose it as a demonic possession case.

Do you personally believe that demonic possession exists?

R: In this Mount Rainier case, it would be difficult, really, to make a case in favor of it. I don't think we can really deny the existence of demonic possession since it is something that we cannot prove nor deny in an indisputable manner. However, to make a case in favor of it, much more evidence is required. Personally, I believe very much in some of the scientific principles often cited in the investigation of anomalistic psychology, among them the Laplace Principle, which indicates that extraordinary claims require extraordinary proof. In this case we don't have that extraordinary proof to make a case in favor of demonic possession. However, I also believe in the principle of Hamlet, which states that all is possible, so there is always a possibility. There is still another principle called the Occam's Razor Principle, which states that when a natural explanation of phenomena in nature is adequate, we don't have to resort to the supernatural. Consequently, in this particular case, I believe that we can account for the case in the context of possible poltergeist phenomena, fraud and psychological mechanism. It seems to me that a mixture of the above hypotheses could very likely explain the phenomena surrounding the Mount Rainier Exorcism. I would sum up the case with the following: that the adolescent made some trickery to cause himself some of the marks that appeared on his body in order to convince his family to allow him to live with his preferred aunt. Therefore, [he did so] to obtain the multiple benefits of avoiding going to school and go to live with his preferred aunt. Basically, poltergeist-like phenomena surround an adolescent who was undergoing some deep-seated stress or psychological conflict, and somehow the stress energy gets transferred outside of the body by some unknown mechanism. I mean that the phenomena may be of a poltergeist nature, but only if the phenomena really took place, as it is reported in the case. The poltergeist hypothesis would also require extraordinary proof to be considered in the top of the hierarchy to explain the phenomena of the case.

Do these phenomena have something to do with the place he was living in?

R: In my opinion, it has nothing to do with the room or the place; it has to do with the person. The poltergeist-like phenomena may come from inside the person, the inner conflict gets out somehow, and it causes the movement of objects and the like. Regarding the poltergeist hypothesis to explain the phenomena, the Reverend Schulze believed to some extent in this hypothesis. Perhaps, the Reverend Schulze was the most objective and scientific person involved in the case, and he witnessed some phenomena that he could not explain. So, I give more weight to his testimony than anybody else's in the Mount Rainier case, because he approached the case with a very scientific mind. Also, I believe most of the parapsychologists may believe that this is a typical conventional poltergeist phenomenon.

Are poltergeist cases very common?

R: Not very common. I mean, there are not many cases reported. There are some studies that have been conducted in that regard to see what is the nature of the phenomena surrounding the poltergeist cases. I have done an evaluation myself of this type of case, a statistical evaluation, for instance comparing cases of poltergeist and demonic possession cases. However, I have found very few differences. Statistically the difference is not significant; they are very similar, except with the religious element that permeates the possession cases. We have found, also, that in many poltergeist cases, trickery has been detected. Some of them are outright trickery and some of them appear to be genuine. Parapsychologists believe some of the phenomena that take place in poltergeist cases are genuine; one the other hand, skeptics believe that trickery takes place in these cases and in all of the cases.

Did the Reverend Schulze publish something on the case?
R: Schulze did not publish anything on the case; however, he was asked to present the case before a parapsychologist association that existed in Washington back then in the 1940s. It was a parapsychology organization and a person who headed the organization was a very close friend of the Reverend Schulze. I think his name was Dick Darnell, who asked him to present the case even before the association. However, he did not want to do that. Even J.B. Rhine, the director of the Duke Parapsychology Laboratory, got caught up in the media with this case, and the media reported that J.B. Rhine had said that the case was one of the most amazing poltergeist cases that that had ever come to his attention.

Did J.B. Rhine as a researcher investigate the case?
R: J.B. Rhine? Well, he didn't really have fully the opportunity to investigate the case, even though he visited the Reverend Schulze at his premises, but the adolescent had been already taken to St, Louis. So he didn't have the opportunity to personally evaluate him. J.B. Rhine considered, however, that very likely it was a case of poltergeist or perhaps the adolescent was playing some tricks to attract attention and to go to go to live with his preferred aunt in St. Louis and avoid schooling.

Who is Dr. J.B. Rhine?
R: Who was J.B. Rhine? Joseph Banks Rhine is considered to be the father of modern experimental parapsychology. He established a parapsychological laboratory at Duke University during the early 1930s. Eventually, the laboratory became the Foundation for Research on the Nature of Man. He did a lot of experimental work using ESP cards to prove that we had capacities of extrasensory perception. He did a lot of work on telepathy and the influence of mind over matter.

How did the Reverend Schulze become interested in parapsychology?
R: He was aware of the work on extrasensory perception that was being carried out by Dr. J.B. Rhine at Duke University. He began to read the books by J.B. Rhine and some of his articles, so that is how he got interested in parapsychology.

Was the Reverend Schulze ever scared about this case?

R: Not at all. He even said at one point that he never sensed a strange presence like a demonic possession presence and the like. This perception of evil is sometimes typical of demonic possession cases that are one of the signs that some experts in demonic possessions believe. It is a symptom of demonic possession, the presence and sensation of some sort of evil on the possessed person.

Was it hard to get the Reverend Schulze to talk to you about the case?

R: It was very difficult because he did not want to reveal any information on the people involved in the case. The Reverend Schulze did not want people to get in trouble because of the press. You know all the press problems; he thought that they were going to go to the media and could distort the facts and affect the people involved in the case. He tried to keep things confidential. Even when I interviewed him, it took me 15 minutes to convince him to talk about the case. Afterwards, he decided to speak to me on the grounds that I was going to use this material only in the context of an academic work or a book, but not for the popular media.

What in your opinion was the process that led a case of poltergeist into one of demonic possession?

R: I believe that when people are undergoing a serious psychological problem, the unconscious mind is very weak and the person becomes very susceptible to suggestions. Now you can imagine in such circumstances what happens if somebody introduces in your mind that you are possessed by the demon and then they proceed to conduct a sophisticated ritual to rid you of the demon. This very impressive ritual, such as an exorcism in which you have to address the Devil directly, you can actually get to the point in your mind that you are really possessed by the Devil. Then the person can begin acting out as if he or she is really possessed. So instead of curing a person, you can create a condition which you are actually trying to avoid. Consequently, I think we should be very careful when diagnosing a case of demonic possession and, also, when you make a decision to perform an exorcism. It is important to note that before we proceed to diagnose a case as a demonic possession case, the Roman Ritual indicates that an exorcist must be able to differentiate between a demonic possession and the symptoms of psychological problems. So we first need to call the judgment of a psychologist or a medical authority. And if a medical doctor and psychologist determine that a person is suffering from a psychological problem, the evangelical authorities should not disagree with the diagnosis. I believe it is healthy for science to keep a balance, on one hand, we have to take into consideration the Laplace principle: that extraordinary claims require extraordinary proof. However, we don't have to close the door for an alternate hypothesis or possibility. Also that there may be other explanations, even though it doesn't fit our current scientific model. We cannot close the door; that is why there is another principle just to keep the balance in science, the Hamlet principle, which states that all is possible. Therefore, we should always leave the door open for an alternate hypothesis or for another possibility. In science, I rather to be critical rather than skeptical. In this particular Mount Rainier case, in spite of my findings that suggest that there may be a natural explanation for the phenomena surrounding the case, however, it took place many years ago, therefore nobody has all the information handy, and thus, we cannot deny in an indisputable manner that the demonic possession case may have taken place, nor that we can explain all the phenomena by the laws of science.

Appendix E

The Documents That Unveil
the Mystery of Ronald's Exorcism

The Jesuit Report or Diary is quite an extensive document, which was sent to Dr. J.B. Rhine, a psychologist at Duke University, for his evaluation by the Rev. Luther Miles Schulze in 1949. This document was found at the archives of the Foundation for Research on the Nature of Man, the foundation that replaced the former Duke Parapsychology Laboratory, which closed in the early 1960s. This document was obtained from the personal correspondence of Dr. J.B. Rhine and Louisa Rhine, housed at the foundation located in Durham, North Carolina. Also, Ida Mae, a personal assistant and secretary of the Reverend Schulze, kept a copy of the Jesuit Report, a copy that she provided for this book.

It is important to note that even though most of the archives of the former Institute of Parapsychology at Duke University became part of Duke's Perkins Library of the University, a lot of the personal correspondence remained at the Foundation for Research on the Nature of Man. Thanks to Anne Carrol, business manager and personal secretary of Dr. J.B. Rhine for over 30 years, the Jesuit Report and other relevant information were found and permission was granted to the author, by Anne Carrol and Richard Broughton (director of research of the Foundation for Research on the Nature of Man), Dr. Ramakrishna Rao (former general director), and John Krugg (current director), to use all the aforementioned documents for the investigation of the Mount Rainier Exorcism for this book. It appears that this document may also have been found by Thomas Allen via alternative sources; he calls it the "Jesuit's Diary," and he uses it as his main source for his book *Possessed*. This document, as the reader may notice, hides the personal information of most of the participants in the events related in it, to maintain their confidentiality. Its contents are included as found in the original document and no editing of it has been conducted to correct mistakes or improve its grammar. Therefore, the reader may find some grammar mistakes; however, the purpose to include it as it is, is to try to provide the reader with a sense of the original document as it was written.

241

CASE STUDY

Birth: 1935
Religion: Evangelical Lutheran; baptized 6 mo. after birth by a Lutheran
Minister
Maternal Grandmother - practicing Catholic until the age of 14 yrs.
Paternal Grandfather - Baptized Catholic but no practice
Father - Baptized Catholic but no instruction or practice
Mother - Baptized Lutheran
Ronald and his mother visited in St. Louis XXXXXXXX at the home of Mr. and
Mrs. XXXXXX.

Background of the Case.

On January 15, 1949, at the home of XXXXXXXX in Cottage City, Maryland a
dripping noise was heard by XXXXXXX and his grandmother in the
grandmother's bedroom. This noise was continued for a short time and then
the picture of Christ on the wall shook as if the wall back of it had been
bumped. By the time the parents of R returned home there was a very definite
scratching sound under the floor boards near the grandmother's bed. From this
night on, the scratching was heard every night about seven o'clock and would
continue until midnight. The family thought that the scratching was caused by
a rodent of some kind. An exterminator was called in who placed chemicals
under the floor boards, but the scratching sound continued and became more
distinct when people stamped on the floor.

This scratching continued for ten days and then stopped. The family finally
believed that the rodent had died. The boy, R, seemed to think he still heard
the noise but the family did not hear anything for a period of three days. When
the sound became audible again, it was no longer in the upstairs bedroom but
had moved downstairs in the boy's bedroom. It was heard as the sound of
squeaking shoes along the bed and was heard at night only when the boy went
to bed. The squeaking sound continued for six nights, and on the sixth night
scratching again was audible. The mother, grandmother and boy while lying
on the bed on this night heard something coming toward them similar to the
rhythm of marching feat and the beat of drums. The sound would travel the
length of the mattress and then back again and repeat this action until the
mother asked, "Is this you, Aunt XXXXXXXX ?" (XXXXXXX had died in St.
Louis two weeks after the first sounds were heard in the home of R.) The
mother continued asking questions but had no verbal reply. She asked this
question, "If you are XXXXXXXX, knock three times." There were waves of air
striking the grandmother, mother and the boy, and three distinct knocks were
heard on the floor. The mother asked again, "If you are XXXXXXXX, tell me
positively by knocking four times." Four distinct knocks were heard. Then
there followed claw scratchings on the mattress.

1

Illustration of the front page of the Jesuit Report (Historical Records, Rhine Research Center 2017, used with permission).

The Jesuit Report is a 29-page document sent to Dr. J.B. Rhine by the Rev. Luther Miles Schulze with a personal letter in 1949. The first section of the document describes a case study in which the general information of the ostensibly possessed adolescent are included: birth date, name of parents, religion, baptized status, religion, etc. In the second section, background information of the case is provided, an account of how all the strange phenomena (possession or poltergeist-like phenomena) began to manifest in this case. In the third section, the author of the document includes one designated "Other manifestations," to describe other phenomena that took place in the case. It is important to note that at the end of the case study section, the actual name of the "possessed" was included. Once the information of the case and the introduction of the phenomena is provided, the author of the Jesuit Report, begins to write the complete story with a dated sequence of events. This strategy of the author to reveal the sequence of events of the Mount Rainier Exorcism is fascinating and historically very important for researchers of this type of demonic possession case, since as far as I know, this would be the most complete actual exorcism case ever documented in the history of demonic possession. The account provides a wealth of information from which the case can be evaluated from a scientific standpoint. Also, to assure the veracity of the events related to the case the diarist was relating, he includes a section on the people who were witnesses to the paranormal events surrounding the adolescent. Moreover, the diarist begins the day-by-day of the events surrounding the exorcism of Ronald on March 7, 1949.

Chapter Notes

Chapter 2

1. J. Nicola, *Diabolical Possession and Exorcism* (Rockford, IL: Tan Books, 1974).

2. Martin Gunther and Berny Brown presented a special report for the *National Tattler* titled "The actual case that became the basis for the movie happened in 1949" and "*The Exorcist* will become the best money maker in movies' history." They both address the issue of the impact of *The Exorcist* on moviegoers.

3. The case is reported A.J.W. Taylor in "Possession and Exorcism," *Expository Times* 76, No. 12 (September 1975).

4. On August 20, 1949, the *Washington Post* published an article by Bill Brinkley titled "Priest Frees Mount Rainier Boy Held in Devil's Grip" (p. 1A).

Chapter 3

1. The investigation of the case by Thomas B. Allen, who found the diary of the Mount Rainier case, is contained in his book *Possessed* (New York: Doubleday, 1993). The research by Dr. Sergio Antonio Rueda was conducted for several years with a research grant from the Parapsychological Foundation of New York.

2. Corrado Balducci, once an official exorcist of the Vatican, one of the best Catholic theologians, has addressed the issue of demonic possession and exorcism. It is considered by demonologists as one of his best books on the topic: *Diavolo: Vivo e Atuante no Mundo* (*The Devil: Alive and Active in Our World*, 1990).

3. William Peter Blatty, *I'll Tell Them I Remember You* (Toronto: George McLeod, 1973).

4. Scott Rogo, *The Poltergeist Experience* (New York: Penguin, 1979).

5. Denis Brian, *Rhine: An Authorized Biography* (Englewood Cliffs, NJ: Prentice-Hall, 1982). Quote by Father William Bowdern is cited by Denis Brian in his book *The Enchanted Voyager: The Life of J.B. Rhine* (p. 183), in which, according to him, the exorcist wrote to William Peter Blatty.

6. Ibid.

7. Le Compte Laplace, *Essai Philosophique sur les Probabilités* (Paris: Mme. V. Courcier, 1814), p. 50.

8. Juan Cortes and Florence Gatti, in their book *The Case Against Possessions and Exorcisms* (New York: Vintage Press, 1975). This anecdotal type of evidence involving parapsychological research is included in J.J. Heaney's book *The Sacred and the Psychic: Parapsychology and Christian Theology* (Ramsey, NJ: Paulist Press, 1984), p. 6.

Chapter 4

1. Letter from the Reverend Luther Miles Schulze, from St. Stephen's Evangelical Church, to Dr. J.B. Rhine. March 21, 1949. Housed at Archives of Perkins Library, Duke University.

2. Letter from Dr. J.B. Rhine, Director of Duke's University Parapsychology Laboratory, to the Reverend Luther Miles Schulze, April 2, 1949. Archives, Perkins Library, Duke University.

3. The Jesuit Report contains the sequence of events of the exorcism practiced on Ronald by the Jesuits. It was sent by the Reverend

Schulze to Dr. J.B. Rhine and reflects the similar content of the so-called Diary that was used by Thomas B. Allen to report his story. The Jesuit Report is mentioned initially by Dr. J.B. Rhine in a letter dated July 1, 1949.

4. In order to protect the identity of some of the participants in this book, in some cases of citations, I will not use their actual names.

5. Allen, *Possessed.*

6. Notes from interview with Ida Mae, one of the most active members of the Reverend Schulze's congregation. I personally interviewed her on July 25, 1990, at the Lutheran Retirement Home. She also guided me on a trip to take a look at the places where most of the events of the Mount Rainier Exorcism had taken place.

7. Notes from the interview that I conducted with the Reverend Luther Miles Schulze at the Lutheran Retirement Home on November 11, 1993, Chevy Chase, MD.

Chapter 5

1. T.K. Oesterreich, *Possession, Demoniacal & Other: Among Primitive Races in Antiquity, the Middle Ages, and Modern Times* (New Hyde Park, NY: University Books, 1966).

2. G. Amorth, *An Exorcist Tells His Story* (San Francisco: Ignatius Press, 1990; original Italian title, *Un escorista raconta*, Rome: Edizioni Dehoniane, 1990).

3. *Ibid.*

4. "Demoniacal Possession," *Catholic Encyclopedia* (New York: Robert Appleton, 1913). See also Louis Jacobs, "Exorcism," *Oxford Reference Online* (Oxford University Press, 1999). Retrieved 24 Jan 2011.

5. Roman Ritual for Use in the United States. Sancta Misa: Rituale Romanun. Canons Regular of St. John Cantius, 1964.

Chapter 10

1. Nicola, *Diabolical Possession and Exorcism.*

2. What Is Occam's Razor? http://math.ucr.edu/home/baez/physics/General/occam.html.

3. How Occam's Razor Works: http://science.howstuffworks.com/innovation/scientific-experiments/occams-razor.htm.

4. Brian, *The Enchanted Voyager.*

5. The investigation of the case by Thomas B. Allen, who found the diary of the Mount Rainier case, is contained in his book *Possessed.* The research by Sergio Rueda was presented at the 49th Annual Convention of the Parapsychological Association. Proceedings of Presented Papers (August 5–6, 2006), Stockholm, Sweden.

Chapter 11

1. R. Thouless, *Experimental Psychical Research* (NJ: Penguin Books, 1963).

2. Brian, *The Enchanted Voyager.*

3. Letter from Dr. J.B. Rhine to the Reverend Luther Miles Schulze, April 2, 1949. Housed at the Archives of the Parapsychology Institute. Duke University.

4. Letter from Dr. J.B. Rhine to the Reverend Luther Miles Schulze, April 21, 1949. Housed at the Archives of the Parapsychology Institute. Duke University.

5. Letter from Dr. J.B. Rhine to the Reverend Luther Miles Schulze, July 1, 1949. Housed at the Archives of the Parapsychology Institute, Duke University.

6. Cortes and Gatti, *The Case Against Possessions and Exorcisms.*

7. Interview with the Reverend Luther Miles Schulze, November 11, 1993.

8. *Ibid.*

9. Jesuit Report, p. 2.

10. Interview with Ida Mae Donley, July 21, 1991.

11. Allen, *Possessed.*

12. Jesuit Report, p. 2.

13. Jesuit Report, p. 2.

14. Jesuit Report, p. 2.

15. *Ibid.*

16. Interview with Jorge Fierro, MD, dermatology specialist, private practice at Cento Médico in Juárez, Mexico, June 23, 2006.

17. S. Lachman, *Psychosomatic Disorders: A Behavioral Interpretation.* Approaches to Behavior Psychology Series (New York: John Wiley & Sons, 1972).

Chapter 12

1. Letter from Luther Miles Schulze to Dr. J.B. Rhine, March 21, 1949. Housed at the Archives of the Institute for Parapsychology, Duke University.

2. *Ibid.*
3. Letter from Richard Darnell, member of the Washington Society for Parapsychology, dated July 5, 1949. Housed at the Archives, Perkins Library, Duke University.
4. *Ibid.*
5. Interview with the Reverend Luther Miles Schulze, November 11, 1993.
6. American Psychiatric Association, *Diagnostic and Statistical Manual of Mental Disorders*, Fourth Edition [DSM-IV] (1994).
7. Lachman, *Psychosomatic Disorders.*
8. Interview with Dr. Jorge Fierro, June 23, 2006.
9. Letter from Luther Miles Schulze to Dr. J.B. Rhine, March 21, 1949. Housed at the Archives Perkins Library, Duke University.
10. Lachman, *Psychosomatic Disorders.*
11. *Ibid.*
12. *Ibid.*
13. Letter from Luther Miles Schulze to Dr. J.B. Rhine, March 21, 1949. Housed at the Archives of Perkins Library, Duke University.
14. *Ibid.*
15. Allen, *Possessed.*

Chapter 13

1. Terence Hines, *Pseudoscience and the Paranormal* (Buffalo, NY: Prometheus Books, 2003), p. 98.
2. Joe Nickell, *The Science of Ghosts: Searching for Spirits of the Dead* (Buffalo, NY: Prometheus Books, 2012), p. 283.
3. Joe Nickell, "Enfield Poltergeist, Investigative Files," August 2012. Committee for Skeptical Inquiry. Retrieved 3 December 2013.
4. R. Lange and J. Houran, "Delusions of the paranormal: A haunting question of perception," *Journal of Nervous and Mental Disease* 186 (10) (1998): pp. 637–645.
5. Joanna Timms, "Phantasm of Freud: Nandor Fodor and the Psychoanalytic Approach to the Supernatural in Interwar Britain," *Psychoanalysis and History* 14:5 (2012).
6. W.G. Roll, *The Poltergeist* (New York: Nelson Doubleday, 1972).
7. Allan Kardec, *Le Livre des Esprits* (France: Editions de Montagne, 2000), chapter 106, "Jean de Bonnot," p. 46.
8. Nicola, *Diabolical Possession and Exorcism.*

9. Letter from Luther Miles Schulze to Dr. J.B. Rhine, March 21, 1949. Housed at the Archives of Perkins Library, Duke University.
10. Brian, *The Enchanted Voyager.*
11. Letter from Dr. J.B. Rhine to the Reverend Luther Miles Schulze, April 2, 1949. Housed at the Archives of Perkins Library. Duke University.
12. *Ibid.*
13. Letter from Dr. J.B. Rhine to the Reverend Luther Miles Schulze, April 21, 1949. Housed at the Archives of Perkins Library, Duke University.
14. Letter from the Reverend Luther Miles Schulze to Dr. J.B. Rhine, July 1, 1949. Housed at the Archives of Perkins Library, Duke University.
15. Letter from the Reverend Luther Miles Schulze to Dr. J.B. Rhine, April 19, 1949. Housed at the Archives of Perkins Library, Duke University.
16. Letter from Dr. J.B. Rhine to the Reverend Luther Miles Schulze, July 1, 1949. Housed at the Archives of Perkins Library, Duke University.
17. Cortes and Gatti, *The Case Against Possessions and Exorcisms.*
18. Brian, *The Enchanted Voyager.*
19. Interview with the Reverend Luther Miles Schulze, November 11, 1993.
20. *Ibid.*
21. *Ibid.*
22. M. Martin, *El rehén del Diablo* (México: Editorial Diana, 1967).
23. Cortes and Gatti, *The Case Against Possessions and Exorcisms.*
24. Letter from Luther Miles Schulze to Dr. J.B. Rhine, September 19, 1949. Housed at the Archives of Perkins Library, Duke University.
25. Letter from Dr. J.B. Rhine to the Reverend Luther Schulze, September 21, 1949. Housed at the Archives of Perkins Library, Duke University.
26. Alan G. Hefner, "Poltergeist," Paranormal encyclopedia.com.
27. B. Shulman, "Adolescence," in R. Corsini, editor, *Encyclopedia of Psychology*, vol. 1 (New York: John Wiley & Sons, 1994).
28. *Ibid.*
29. Letter from the Reverend Luther Schulze to Dr. J.B. Rhine, September 19, 1949. Housed at the Archives of the Institute for Parapsychology, Duke University.
30. E.H. Erikson, *Childhood and Society* (New York: Norton, 1950).

31. Ida Mae Donley, interviews, July 25, 1991, and November 11, 1993, at the Lutheran Retirement Home and at her home.

32. A. Gauld and A.D. Cornell, *Poltergeists* (Boston: Routledge & Kegan Paul, 1979).

33. W.G. Roll, "Poltergeists," in B.B. Wolman, ed., *Handbook of Parapsychology* (New York: Van Nostrand Reinhold, 1977), pp. 382–413.

34. Rogo, *The Poltergeist Experience*.

35. Allen, *Possessed*.

36. Rogo, *The Poltergeist Experience*.

37. H.J. Irwin, *Psi and the Mind: An Information Processing Approach* (Metuchen, NJ: Scarecrow Press, 1979).

38. J. Palmer, "A case of RSPK involving a ten-year old boy: the Powhatan poltergeist," *Journal of the American Society for Psychical Research* 68 (1974): pp. 1–33.

39. J.G. Pratt and J. Palmer, "An investigation of an unpublicized family poltergeist," in J.D. Morris, W.G. Roll, and R.L. Morris, eds., *Research in Parapsychology 1976* (Metuchen, NJ: Scarecrow Press, 1976).

40. Roll, "Poltergeists."

41. Gauld and Cornell, *Poltergeists*.

42. *Ibid.*

43. Roll, "Poltergeists."

44. *Ibid.*

45. Rogo, *The Poltergeist Experience*.

46. H. Bender, "New developments in poltergeist research," *Proceedings of the Parapsychological Association* 6 (1969): pp. 81–109.

47. J. Mischo, "Personality structure of psychokinetic mediums," *Proceedings of the Parapsychological Association* 5 (1968): pp. 38–37.

48. A.R.G. Owen, *Can We Explain the Poltergeist?* (New York: Garrett, 1964).

49. Irwin, *Psi and the mind*.

50. Rogo, *The Poltergeist Experience*.

51. Heaney, *The Sacred and the Psychic*.

52. Rogo, *The Poltergeist Experience*. New York: Penguin.

53. Oesterreich, *Possession, Demoniacal & Other*.

54. *Ibid.*

55. H. Thurston, *Ghosts and Poltergeists* (London: Burns, Oates, 1953).

Chapter 14

1. John Warwick Montgomery, "Exorcism: Is it for real?" *Christianity Today*, July 26, 1974.

2. Fr. Gabriel Amorth, *The Real Exorcist* (Ft. Collins, CO: Ignatius Press, 1974). The Chief Exorcist of the Vatican tells his story as an exorcist.

3. *Ibid.*

4. Brian, *The Enchanted Voyager*, p. 183.

5. Nicola, *Diabolical Possession and Exorcism*.

6. Allen, *Possessed*.

7. Cortes and Gatti, *The Case Against Possessions and Exorcisms*.

8. Balducci, *Diavolo*.

9. The Roman Ritual, translated by Philip T. Weller, STD.

10. *Ibid.*

11. Laurie Goldstein, "For Catholics, Interest in Exorcism is Revived," *New York Times*, November 13, 2010.

12. O.G. Quevedo, *Antes que os demonios voltem (Before the Demons Turn Back)* (São Paulo: Ediciones Loyola, 1989).

13. *Ibid.*

14. Dr. Jorge Fierro, a certified dermatologist in private practice in México.

15. Jeff Durmann, book review of Ian Wilson's *The Bleeding Mind: An Investigation of Stigmata* (UK: Paladin Grafton Books, 1991).

16. Letter from Luther Miles Schulze to Dr. J.B. Rhine, March 21, 1949. Housed at the Archives of Perkins Library, Duke University.

17. Interview with the Reverend Luther Miles Schulze, November 11, 1993.

18. Gunther and Brown, "The actual case that became the basis for the movie happened in 1949."

19. Allen, *Possessed*.

20. Oesterreich, *Possession, Demoniacal & Other*.

21. A. Rodewyk, *Possessed by Satan* (New York: Doubleday, 1975).

22. *Ibid.*

23. Quevedo, *Antes que os demonios voltem*.

24. William Sargant, *The Mind Possessed: A Physiology of Possession, Mysticism and Faith Healing* (New York: Harper and Row, 1974).

25. Oesterreich, *Possession, Demoniacal & Other*.

26. Brinkley, "Priest Frees Mount Rainier Boy Held in Devil's Grip."

27. Jeremiah O'Leary, "The Exorcist: Story That Almost Wasn't," *Washington Star-News*, December 29, 1973.

28. O.G. Quevedo, *El rostro oculto de la mente* (*The Concealed Face of The Mind*) (Spain: Sal Terrae, 1974).

29. *Ibid.*

30. J.M. Heredia, *Spiritism and Common Sense* (New York: P.J. Kenedy, 1922).

31. C. Richet, *Traité de métapsychique* (Paris: F. Alcan, 1922).

32. Quevedo, *Antes que os demonios voltem.*

Chapter 15

1. Letter from the Reverend Luther Schulze, to Dr. J.B. Rhine, March 21, 1949. Housed at the Archived of Perkins Library, Duke University.

2. *Ibid.*

3. Interview (part 2) with Luther Miles Schulze, November 11, 1993.

4. Letter from Dr. J.B. Rhine to the Reverend Luther Miles Schulze, April 21, 1949. Duke University, Archives Perkins Library.

5. Letter from Richard Darnell to Dr. J.B. Rhine, May 17, 1949, Duke University, Perkins Library.

6. Letter from Luther Miles Schulze to Dr. J.B Rhine, April 6, 1949. Duke University, Perkins Library.

7. Letter from the Reverend Luther Schulze to Dr. J.B. Rhine, March 21, 1949. Housed at the Archived of Perkins Library, Duke University.

8. *Ibid.*

9. Letter from the Reverend Luther Schulze to Dr. J.B. Rhine, April 19, 1949. Housed at the Archives of Perkins Library, Duke University.

10. *Ibid.*

11. Letter from the Reverend Luther Schulze to Dr. J.B. Rhine, September 19, 1949. Housed at the Archives of Perkins Library, Duke University.

12. Letter from the Reverend Luther Schulze to Dr. J.B Rhine, April 19, 1949.

13. Letter from Richard Darnell to Dr. J.B. Rhine, June 7, 1949. Duke University, Perkins Library.

14. Letter from Richard Darnell to Dr. J.B. Rhine, July 5, 1949, Duke University, Perkins Library.

15. Letter from Dr. J.B. Rhine to the Reverend Luther Miles Schulze, June 7, 1949. Duke University, Archives, Perkins Library.

16. Letter from Dr. J.B. Rhine to Dick Darnell, August 17, 1949, Duke University, Perkins Library.

Chapter 16

1. M. Brownwell, "Demonic Possession," on Serendip: 1999 Final Web Reports (2008).

2. Letter from the Reverend Luther Schulze to Dr. J.B. Rhine, September 19, 1949. Housed at the Archives of Perkins Library, Duke University.

3. Letter from the Reverend Luther Schulze to Dr. J.B. Rhine, March 21, 1949. Housed at the Archives of Perkins Library, Duke University.

4. *Ibid.*

5. Report of the Mount Rainier case from the Reverend Luther Schulze to Dr. J.B. Rhine, March 21, 1949. Archives, Perkins Library, Duke University.

6. Allen, *Possessed.*

7. C. Balducci, *Diavolo.*

8. Montgomery, "Exorcism: Is it for real?"

9. Quevedo, *El rostro oculto de la mente.*

10. Nicola, *Diabolical Possession.*

11. Cardinal Jorge Medina Estevez, "Demonic Possession & Oppression and Exorcism: Roman Catholic Beliefs and Practices." Religious Tolerance.org, 1998–2010, p. 1. Ontario Consultants on Religious Tolerance.

12. Brownwell, "Demonic Possession."

Sources

Allen, T.B. 1993. *Possessed: The True Story of an Exorcism*. New York: Doubleday.

American Psychiatric Association. 1994. *Diagnostic and Statistical Manual of Mental Disorders*, fourth edition. Arlington, VA: American Psychiatric Association.

Amorth, G. 1974. *The Real Exorcist*. Ft. Collins, CO: Ignatius Press.

_____. 1990. *An Exorcist Tells His Story*. Ft. Collins, CO: Ignatius Press. Originally published in Italian as *Un escorista raconta*, Rome: Edizioni Dehoniane, 1990.

Balducci, C. 1990. *Diavolo: vivo e atuante no mundo* (*The Devil: Alive and Active in Our World*). New York: Alba House.

Barrett, W. 1926. *Death-Bed Visions*. London: Methuen.

Bender, H. 1969. New Developments in Poltergeist Research. *Proceedings of the Parapsychological Association*. Parapsychological Association.

Blatty, W. 1971. *The Exorcist*. New York: Bantam.

_____. 1973. *I'll Tell Them I Remember You*. Toronto: George McLeod.

Bozzuto, J. 1975. Cinematic Neurosis Following *The Exorcist*: Report of Four Cases. *Journal of Nervous and Mental Disease* 161 (1): 43–48.

Brian, D. 1982. *Rhine: An Authorized Biography*. Englewood Cliffs, NJ: Prentice-Hall.

Brinkley, B. 1949, August 20. Priest Frees Mount Rainier Boy Held in Devil's Grip. *Washington Post*, p. 1A.

Brown, B., and M. Gunther. 1973. The Actual Case That Became the Basis for the Movie Happened in 1949. *National Tattler*.

_____. 1974. *The Exorcist* Will Become the Best Money Maker in Movies' History. *National Tattler*, Special Edition, p. 1.

Brownwell, M. 2008, January 4. Serendip Studio. Retrieved April 23, 2010, from http://serendip.brynmawr.edu/exchange/serendipupdate/demonic-possession.

Cantius, C.R. 2010. Roman Ritual for Use in the United States. Sancta Misa: Rituale Romanum. Chicago, Illinois.

Cardeña, E., S.J. Lynn, and Stanley Krippner, eds. 2000. *Varieties of Anomalous Experience: Examining the Scientific Evidence*. Washington, D.C.: American Psychological Association.

Darnell, R. 1949, May 17. Letter to Dr. J.B. Rhine. Washington, D.C.: Washington Society for Parapsychology.

_____. 1949, June 7. Letter to Dr. J.B. Rhine. Washington, D.C.: Washington Society for Parapsychology.

_____. 1949, July 5. Letter. Washington, D.C.: Washington Society for Parapsychology.

_____. 1949, July 5. Letter. Washington, D.C.: Archives Duke University: Perkins Library.

Demoniacal Possession (1913). *Catholic Encyclopedia*. New York: Robert Appleton.

Donley, Ida Mae. 1990. Interview. Lutheran Retirement Home, Chevy Chase, MA.

Durmann, J. 1991. Book review of Ian Wilson's *The Bleeding Mind: An Investigation of Stigmata*. UK: Paladin Grafton Books.

Erikson, E.H. 1950. *Childhood and Society.* New York: Norton.
Estevez, Cardinal J.M. 1998–2010. Demonic possession & oppression; exorcism: Roman Catholic beliefs and practices. Tolerance.org.
Gatti, F., and J. Cortes. 1975. *The Case Against Possessions and Exorcisms.* New York: Vintage Press.
Gauld, A., and A.D. Cornell. 1979. *Poltergeists.* Boston: Routledge & Kegan Paul.
Ghosts and Poltergeists. 1953. London: Burns, Oates.
Goodman, L., and A. Gilman. 1975. *The Pharmacological Basis of Therapeutics.* New York: Macmillan.
Goldstein, L. 2010, November 12. For Catholics, interest in exorcism is revived. *New York Times.*
Heaney, J. 1984. *The Sacred and the Psychic: Parapsychology and Christian Theology.* New York: Paulist Press.
Hefner, A.G. 2008, June 28. Paranormal encyclopedia.com. Retrieved June 23, 2016, from http://www.paranormal-encyclopedia.com/p/poltergeist/.
Heredia, J. 1922. *Spiritism and Common Sense.* New York: P.J. Kenedy.
Hines, T. 2003. *Pseudoscience and the Paranormal.* Buffalo, NY: Prometheus Books.
Houran, J., and R. Lange. 1998. Delusions of the Paranormal: A Haunting Question of Perception. *Journal of Nervous and Mental Disease* 186 (10) (1998): pp. 637–645.
Irwin, H. 1979. *Psi and the Mind: An Information Processing Approach.* Metuchen, NJ: Scarecrow Press.
Jesuit Report. 1949. Archives, Institute for Parapsychology/Rhine Research Foundation. Durham, NC.
Kardec, A. 1990. *Le livre des esprits.* France: Editions de Montagne.
Krippner, S. 1997. Dissociation in Many Times and Places. In S. Krippner and S.M. Powers, eds., *Broken Images, Broken Selves: Dissociative Narratives in Clinical Practice.* Washington, D.C.: Brunner Mazel.
Lachman, S. 1972. *Psychosomatic Disorders: A Behavioral Interpretation.* Approaches to Behavioral Psychology Series. New York: John Wiley & Sons.
Long, J. 1977. *The Essential Guide to Prescription Drugs.* New York: HarperCollins.
Martin, M. 1967. *El rehén del diablo.* México, DF: Diana.
Martinez Taboas, A. 1980. The Psychological Model of Poltergeist Phenomena: Some Criticisms and Suggestions. *Parapsychology Review* 11(2), 24–27.
McManus, J., ed. *Mysteries of the Unknown.* Alexandria, VA: Time-Life Books.
Mischo, J. 1969. Personality Structure of Psychokinetic Mediums. Proceedings of the Parapsychological Association (pp. 5, 38–37). Parapsychological Association.
Montgomery, J.W. July 26, 1974. Exorcism: Is it for Real? *Christianity Today.*
"New Advent" (1913). *Catholic Encyclopedia.* Retrieved June 20, 2010, from http://www.newadvent.org/cathen/12315a.htm.
Nickell, J. 2012. Enfield Poltergeist, Investigative Files. *Skeptical Enquirer.*
_____. 2012. *The Science of Ghosts: Searching for Spirits of the Dead.* Buffalo, NY: Prometheus.
Nicola, J. 1974. *Diabolical Possession and Exorcism.* Rockford, IL: Tan Books.
Oesterreich, T.K. 1966. *Possession, Demoniacal & Other: Among Primitive Races in Antiquity, the Middle Ages, and Modern Times.* New Hyde Park, NY: University Books.
O'Leary, J. 1973, 29 December. The Exorcist: The Story That Almost Wasn't. *Washington Star-News.*
Owen, A.R. 1964. *Can We Explain the Poltergeist?* New York: Garrett.
Palmer, J. 1974. A Case of RSPK Involving a Ten-Year-Old Boy: The Powhatan Poltergeist. *Journal of the American Society for Psychical Research* 68, 1–33.
Pratt, J.G., and J. Palmer. 1976. An Investigation of an Unpublicized Family Poltergeist. In J.D. Morris, W.G. Roll, and R.L. Morris, eds., *Research in Parapsychology 1976.* Metuchen, NJ: Scarecrow Press.
Quevedo, O.G, 1974. *El rostro oculto de la mente (The concealed face of the mind).* Spain: Sal Terrae.

_____. 1989. *Antes que os Demonios Voltem (Before the Demons Turn Back)*. São Paulo: Ediciones Loyola.

Rhine, J.B. 1949, April 2. Letter to Luther Miles Schulze. Durham, NC: Archives, Perkins Library, Duke University.

_____. 1949, April 19. Letter to Reverend Luther Miles Schulze. Durham, NC.

_____. 1949, April 21. Letter to Reverend Luther Miles Schulze. Durham, NC.

_____. 1949, June 7. Letter to Reverend Luther Miles Schulze. Durham, NC: Archives, Perkins Library, Duke University.

_____. 1949, July 1. Letter to Reverend Luther Miles Schulze. Durham, NC.

_____. 1949, August 17. Letter to Richard Darnell. Durham, NC: Archives, Perkins Library, Duke University.

_____. 1949, September 21. Letter to Reverend Luther Schulze. Durham, NC: Archives, Perkins Library, Duke University.

Richet, C 1922. *Traité de métapsychique*. Paris: F. Alcan

Rodewyk, A. 1975. *Possessed by Satan*. New York: Doubleday.

Rogo, S. 1978. *Minds in Motion: The Riddle of Psychokinesis*. New York: Taplinger.

_____. 1979. *The Poltergeist Experience*. New York: Penguin.

Roll, W.G. 1972. *The Poltergeist*. New York: Nelson Doubleday.

_____. 1977. Poltergeists. In B.B. Wolman, ed., *Handbook of Parapsychology*. New York: Van Nostrand Reinhold.

Roman Catholic Church. 2007. Roman Ritual: Christian Burial and Office for the Dead, Exorcism, Blessings Reserved to Religious or to Certain Places, vol. 2. Preserving Christian Publications.

Rueda, S. November 11, 1990. Notes from interview with the Reverend Luther Miles Schulze at the Lutheran Retirement Home. Chevy Chase, MD.

_____. November 11, 1990. Notes from interview with Ida Mae Donley. Rockville, MD.

_____. July 25, 1993. Notes from interview with the Reverend Luther Miles Schulze at the Lutheran Retirement Home. Chevy Chase, MD.

_____. June 23, 2006. Interview with Jorge Fierro, MD, dermatology specialist. Cd. Juárez, Chihuahua, México.

_____. 2006. A Medical-Psychological Approach to the Possession Case Behind William Blatty's The Exorcist. The Parapsychological Association 49th Annual Convention Proceedings of Presented Papers (pp. 216–224). Stockholm, Sweden: The Parapsychological Association.

Sargant, W. 1974. *The Mind Possessed: A Physiology of Possession, Mysticism and Faith Healing*. New York: Harper & Row.

Schulze, L.M. 1949, March 21. Letter to Dr. J.B. Rhine. Washington, D.C.: Archives, Perkins Library, Duke University.

_____. 1949, March 21. Report of the Mount Rainier case. Washington, DC: Archives, Perkins Library, Duke University.

_____. 1949, April 2. Letter to Dr. J.B Rhine. Washington, D.C.: Archives, Perkins Library, Duke University.

_____. 1949, April 6. Letter to Dr. J.B Rhine. Washington, D.C.: Archives, Perkins Library, Duke University.

_____. 1949, April 19. Letter to Dr. J.B Rhine. Washington, D.C.: Archives, Perkins Library, Duke University.

_____. 1949, July 21. Letter to Dr. J.B. Rhine, Washington, D.C. Archive, Perkins Library, Duke University.

_____. 1949, September 19. Letter to Dr. J.B. Rhine. Washington, D.C.: Archive, Perkins Library, Duke University.

Shulman, B. "Adolescence." In R. Corsini, ed. (1994). *Encyclopedia of Psychology*, vol. 1. New York: John Wiley & Sons.

Taylor, A. 1975. Possession and Exorcism. *Expository Times* 76, No. 12.

Thornburn, W.M. 1915. Occam's Razor. *Mind* 24, pp. 287–288.

Thouless, R. 1963. *Experimental Psychical Research*. NJ: Penguin Books.
Timms, J. 2012. Phantasm of Freud: Nandor Fodor and the Psychoanalytic Approach to the Supernatural in Interwar. *Psychoanalysis and History* 14:5.
What Is Occam's Razor? 1997. Retrieved March 6, 2011, from http://math.ucr.edu/home/baez/physics/General/occam.html.

Index